the *natural* menopause cookbook

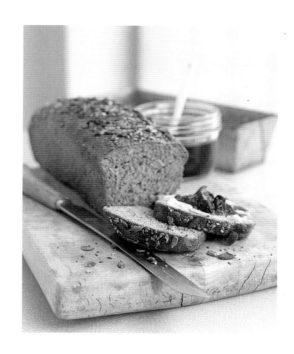

the *natural* menopause cookbook

Ease your symptoms with over 70 delicious recipes

Angie Jefferson and Fiona Hunter

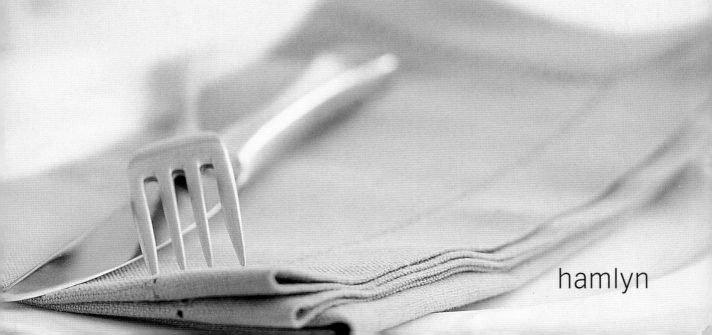

hamlyn

First published in Great Britain in 2004 by
Hamlyn, a division of Octopus Publishing Group Ltd
2–4 Heron Quays, London E14 4JP

Distributed in the United States and Canada by Sterling Publishing Co., Inc.
387 Park Avenue South, New York, NY 10016-8810

ISBN 0 600 61097 7

A CIP catalog record for this book is available from the British Library

Printed in China

10 9 8 7 6 5 4 3 2 1

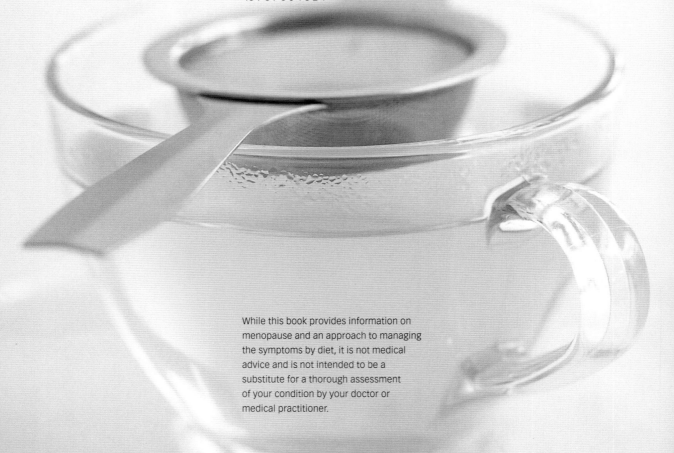

While this book provides information on menopause and an approach to managing the symptoms by diet, it is not medical advice and is not intended to be a substitute for a thorough assessment of your condition by your doctor or medical practitioner.

contents

6   introduction

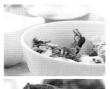

28   breakfasts

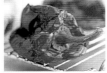

44   light bites

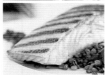

74   main dishes

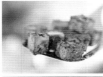

94   vegetarian dishes

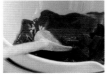

110   desserts

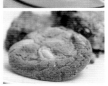

126   baking

144   index and acknowledgements

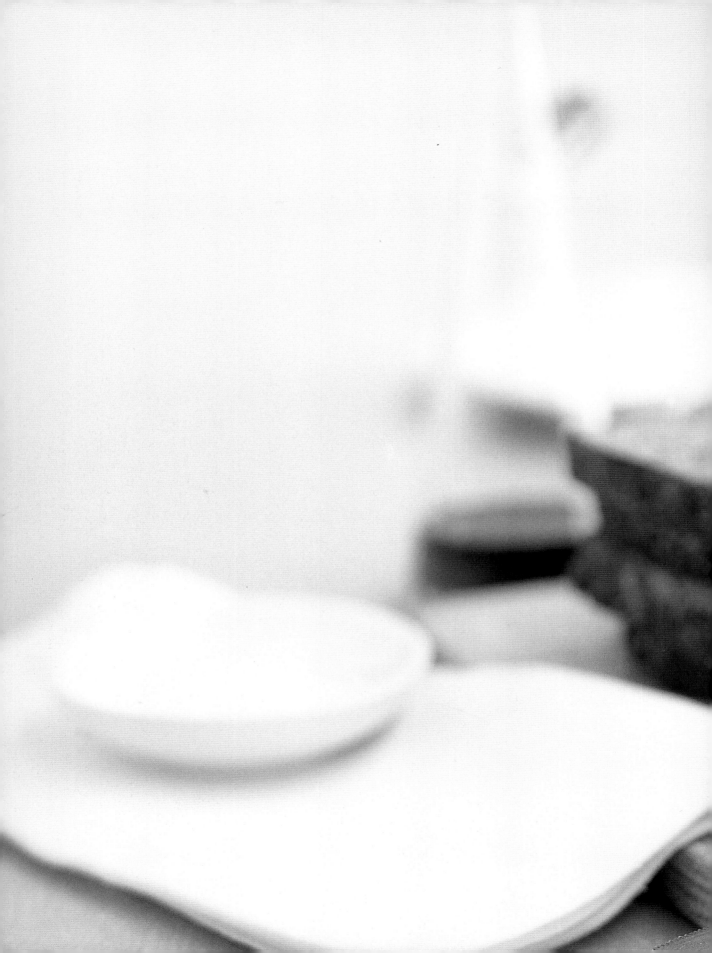

introduction

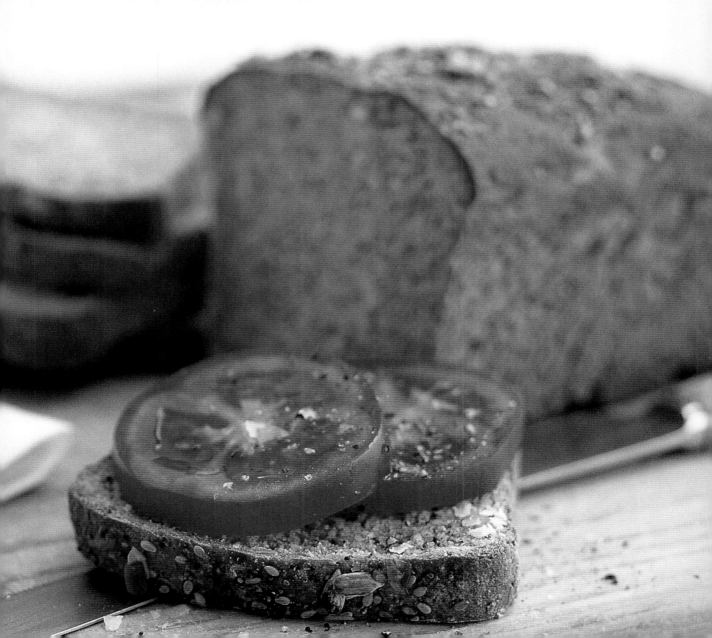

About this book

Menopause can be a time of confusion and mixed emotions. Unsure of what is happening to our bodies, and bombarded with conflicting stories about hormone replacement therapy (HRT), most of us find it difficult to get practical and accurate information. This book provides a simple and down-to-earth approach to the menopausal years and offers advice on how to take control of any troublesome symptoms before they take control of you. In the following pages you will find the information you need to manage the symptoms and effects of menopause, both today and in the years to come.

Menopause is a natural part of a woman's life, signaling an end to her fertile years. While some women sail through it with little difficulty, others experience a range of symptoms, which vary in severity from mild to completely disrupting. Over the past decade HRT has increased in popularity and is used successfully by many, both to treat symptoms and provide health benefits. However, there are health concerns regarding HRT—some women cannot use it and others simply would prefer not to. But HRT is not the only approach available; changing your diet can offer an effective, alternative management strategy.

This book has been written for all menopausal women, whatever their symptoms, and whether or not they are taking HRT. It does not matter whether you are just entering menopause or have been experiencing its effects for some time. The information here will allow you to get the best you can from what you eat, and help alleviate common symptoms.

First we review the changes that are happening to you, and common symptoms and effects arising from these. We then look at healthy eating during menopause, managing your weight, and specific areas of the diet from which you can gain the most benefit. The main section of the book brings your new diet to life with a wide range of tasty and enjoyable recipes.

As with any new diet, the body may require some time to adjust to the changes that you are making and you may not appreciate the full benefits for several months. Be patient and persevere—the boost to your overall health will help you get through menopause with ease.

What is menopause?

Menopause is defined by those in the medical profession as the final menstrual period, and signals the end of a woman's fertility. However, the term is more commonly used to describe the time leading up to the final menstrual period and the time beyond.

For most women, the start of menopause is signaled by their periods becoming increasingly irregular, until they eventually stop. Menopause is considered to be over when no periods have occurred for a year.

The average age that women go through this change is 51 years, but it can occur at any time between the ages of 45 and 55. It is considered premature if it occurs before the age of 40, something which is thought to affect 1 in 100 women. It may also be suddenly induced at any age as a result of illness or a medical procedure, such as a hysterectomy, where the ovaries are removed.

What causes it?

Menopause occurs when your ovaries simply run out of the eggs they release each month during your fertile years. Before puberty the ovaries are packed with eggs and during a woman's life around 450 of them mature and are released to travel down the fallopian tubes and into the womb. This is ovulation. If the egg does not become fertilized, it will pass out of the body along with the womb lining (menstruation). The menstrual cycle is under the control of hormones, and these cause an egg to be released each month and prepare the body for possible fertilization. One of the main hormones is estrogen, which is produced by the ovaries themselves.

Around the age of 45, few eggs remain and the ovaries start to reduce their production of the hormone estrogen, until it stops altogether during the menopausal years. During this time the female body has to adapt from a life that has been dominated by estrogen and the menstrual cycle, to a life without this hormone. It is this decline in estrogen that results in the symptoms many women suffer.

Menopause: ceasing of menstruation; period in a woman's life when this occurs.
Oxford English Dictionary

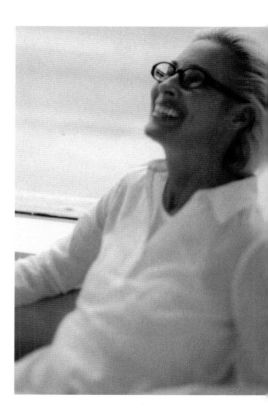

above Changing diet can help to manage menopause.

How do women react?

How women experience menopause depends on several factors, including their diet and nutrition, their general fitness, and physical health, and may even be influenced by women's beliefs and attitudes toward menopause.

What are the symptoms?

Early physical symptoms	Emotional symptoms	Later physical symptoms
Hot flashes	Mood swings and irritability	Dry skin
Night sweats	Inability to cope	Vaginal dryness
Headaches	Lowered self-esteem	Frequent and/or painful urination
Tiredness	Loss of concentration and short-term memory	Stress or urge incontinence
Insomnia		Loss of libido
General aches	Anxiety and depression	Painful sexual intercourse

Menopausal symptoms can last for just a few months or linger for several years. It is estimated that three-quarters of Western women experience one or more of the common symptoms associated with menopause, and that for one-third of those women the symptoms experienced are severe.

Commonly used terms
- Premenopausal—usually a woman in her mid forties who is on the cusp of the menopause.
- Perimenopausal—a woman who is in the midst of menopause.
- Postmenopausal—a woman who has been period-free for at least a year.

Long-term effects of menopause

In the long term, the changing estrogen levels in the body have far-reaching effects on the bones, heart, and blood vessels. Estrogen has a protective effect over the heart, arteries, and veins, and helps promote bone density.

As estrogen levels decline, the risk of developing osteoporosis or heart disease increases significantly. By the age of 50, one in three women are affected by osteoporosis, and almost one-third of premature deaths in women are due to heart disease.

Hormone Replacement Therapy (HRT)

HRT can help alleviate the symptoms of menopause. As the name suggests, it replaces the hormones that are no longer produced by the body—this includes both estrogen and another hormone, progesterone. There are many different combinations and strengths of HRT, and different modes of delivery, including tablets, patches, gels, and implants. Some continue to give a period every month, others every three months, and some no periods at all. Each woman needs to be individually assessed by their doctor to decide which preparation is the right one for them.

below HRT is highly effective, but not the choice of all women.

Pros and cons of HRT

HRT helps to relieve symptoms such as hot flashes, night sweats, and vaginal dryness. It may also offer some protection against heart disease, osteoporosis, and Alzheimer's, although in order to gain most benefit for these conditions, HRT needs to be taken for at least 5–10 years.

However, as with any drug treatment, HRT also holds some negative effects, which include an increased chance of breast cancer and deep vein thrombosis. As we have already seen, HRT is thought to protect women against heart disease, but recent evidence has suggested that specific types of HRT may actually increase the risk. Current advice by the British Heart Foundation (2003) is that women should not take HRT just to avoid heart problems.

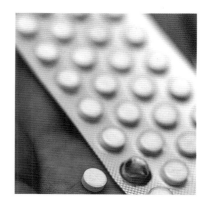

It is important for all women to weigh up the benefits and drawbacks that come with HRT. Make your decision with the help of your doctor to ensure that you are making the best choice for your health.

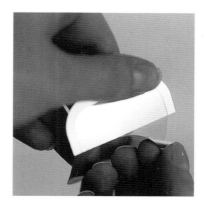

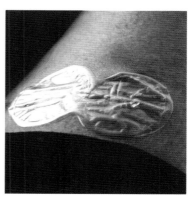

Phytoestrogens—nature's choice

Phytoestrogens are chemicals found in some plants, and are very similar in structure to the human hormone estrogen. Phytoestrogens appear to promote the effects of estrogen in some parts of the body. Studies suggest that eating a diet rich in these plant chemicals holds the potential to alleviate some menopausal symptoms, and may also help to prevent the development of breast cancer, osteoporosis, and heart disease. A phytoestrogen-rich diet offers benefits for men too, protecting the bones, heart, and circulation, and reducing the risk of developing cancer of the prostate. One of the richest sources of phytoestrogens is the soybean, and foods made from this bean (tofu, soy milk, soy yogurts, and so on). They are also found in other beans, linseeds (flaxseeds), and rye. How effective they are will depend on how often you eat them, and how much you have.

below Linseed (flaxseed) is a rich source of phytoestrogens and delicious if toasted and sprinkled over cereal or salads.

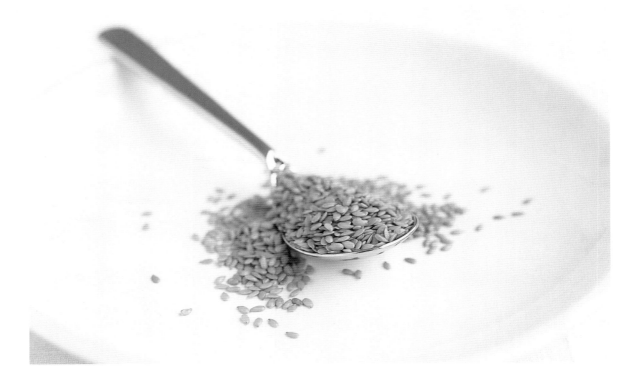

Compared to HRT, phytoestrogens provide much less estrogen, but they can help to counteract the fall in levels around the time of menopause. Phytoestrogens appear to actually reduce the effects of estrogen in certain parts of the body, however. This is believed to be down to different types of body cell receptors for estrogen. Estrogen receptors sit on the outside surfaces of cells and act like lock-and-key mechanisms, allowing the cell to react to estrogen and phytoestrogens. One specific group of receptors, known as alpha-receptors, occur mainly on the sexual organs such as the uterus, ovaries, and breasts, and these respond strongly to estrogen and weakly to phytoestrogens. The other type, beta-estrogen receptors, are more common on bones and blood vessels, and these react more strongly to phytoestrogens.

Phytoestrogens in the diet

There are various different types of phytoestrogens, which are found in different foods, and isoflavones are found in the most commonly eaten foods. The average intake of phytoestrogens in a Western diet is estimated to be just 1–2 mg per day. This may be slightly higher among people eating vegetarian diets containing lots of beans and legumes. Women in Japan and other Eastern countries eat 50–100 mg per day, the amount shown by scientists to provide health benefits.

The great news is that foods that are rich in phytoestrogens are all extremely good for us anyway, containing protein, dietary fiber, and a wide range of vitamins and minerals. Even if we disregard the potential benefits from phytoestrogens, these foods are all well worth including in a healthy balanced diet.

Phytoestrogens and where to find them

Phytoestrogen type	Where they are found
Isoflavones	Peas, beans, soybeans and soy products, lentils, chickpeas
Coumestans	Sprouting beans, such as clover or alfalfa sprouts
Lignans	Linseeds, rye; small amounts in most other cereals, fruit, and vegetables
Prenylated Flavenoids	Hops—some beers

Phytoestrogens and hot flashes

Menopause is much less of a problem in countries where a soy-based diet is eaten, such as Japan and China. In Europe, 80 percent of menopausal women suffer from hot flashes, compared to 57 percent in Malaysia and just 18 percent in China. For one-third of women in Western countries, for example, hot flashes are frequent and severe, and may be accompanied by other symptoms such as headaches, irritability, and tiredness. In Japan, hot flashes are so rare that there are no words to describe this experience in the Japanese language.

However, Japanese women still have menopausal symptoms and report an increase in back and neck aches. It may be that a phytoestrogen-rich diet changes the symptoms of menopause, or that Western women do in fact experience the same symptoms, but are more aware of the problems associated with hot flashes.

below Alfalfa sprouts are a useful source of phytoestrogens and great in salads.

bottom Some traditionally brewed beers contain phytoestrogens.

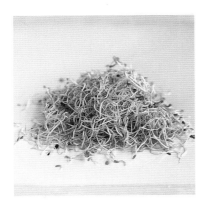

The evidence

Most studies have shown that eating phytoestrogen-rich soy over a 2–3 month period can reduce the frequency and severity of hot flashes. In the main, trials have shown a significant impact when 40–80 mg of phytoestrogens are consumed per day. However, there have also been studies where no effects have been found. The greatest benefits will occur if at present you eat little soy, if your hot flashes are severe, and if you start to eat at least 45 mg every day.

Soy, cholesterol, and heart disease

The death rate from heart disease in Eastern countries, such as Japan and China, is six times lower than death rates in Western countries, such as the USA and the UK. The incidence of heart disease is also lower among vegetarians and vegans than those who eat meat. While many factors are likely to play a part, it is believed that a high intake of soy is one of the factors protecting the heart in Asian and vegetarian diets.

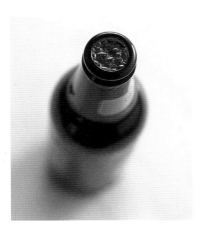

Soy protein, soy fiber, and soy phytoestrogens are all known to have a positive influence over the heart, helping to lower the fat content of the diet, lower cholesterol levels, prevent cholesterol from being deposited into blood vessel walls, and lower blood pressure. If you include soy foods regularly in your diet, you will be gaining all these benefits at once.

How much do I need?

Scientific studies have shown that by eating 25 g of soy protein every day you can lower your cholesterol levels by up to 10 percent. To get 25 g of soya protein, you need to eat around three servings of a soy-based food.

This also happens to be the same amount you need to provide 45 mg of phytoestrogens per day—the amount necessary to relieve hot flashes. Each of your three servings must provide a minimum of 6.25 g of soy protein, which needs to retain its naturally occurring phytoestrogens (see page 17).

Phytoestrogens and osteoporosis

Osteoporosis is a condition caused by loss of bone mineral, resulting in bones that are weak, fragile, and extremely vulnerable to fracture. A range of factors are required to maintain good bone health, one of which is estrogen. The decline in estrogen levels during menopause leads to an increase in the normal rate of mineral loss from bone, and as a result makes postmenopausal women much more vulnerable to osteoporosis.

HRT is known to be effective in preventing osteoporosis, but women consuming diets rich in soy products also have a much-reduced incidence of osteoporosis, suggesting a role for phytoestrogens in preserving bone health.

The evidence

Studies seem to suggest that postmenopausal women who are given phytoestrogen-rich soy have better bone density. The amounts consumed have been in the range of 45–90 mg of phytoestrogens per day, and better effects usually result from higher intakes.

So far, most studies have only lasted six months, whereas any significant improvements in bone structure take around two years. The main benefits have been seen in the spine, which is not surprising as bone "turnover" here is much quicker than in other parts of the body. It is assumed that, given enough time, beneficial effects would be seen in the hips as well. However, the long-term effects of phytoestrogens on bone health still remain to be explored.

Making claims

Since 2002, manufacturers of soy products in the USA and UK have been able to make a health claim on their packaging that "including at least 25 g per day of soy protein as part of a diet low in saturated fat can help to reduce blood cholesterol."

Words of caution about phytoestrogens

It would be naïve to assume that consuming high doses of any substance is always beneficial, and phytoestrogens are no exception. Evidence suggests that the benefits from both phytoestrogens and soy are far greater if they are derived from natural foods (as nature intended and where overdosing is less likely) rather than from concentrated supplements.

One group of women who should exercise caution are those who have breast cancer. Cancerous cells in the breast are generally stimulated by estrogen, and it is unclear at present as to whether phytoestrogens stimulate or inhibit these cells. Research is underway to answer this question.

Some experts believe that food-derived phytoestrogens do not present a risk to those with breast cancer, but do not recommend phytoestrogen supplements for these women. Other experts believe that phytoestrogens from any source can be damaging to women with breast cancer. Until we have a definite answer it is prudent to be cautious and for those affected not to increase their intake of phytoestrogens, either by diet or supplementation.

A second group who should be aware of the potential effects of a higher phytoestrogen intake are women taking thyroxine. Phytoestrogens may affect thyroxine replacement therapy. If you increase your intake of phytoestrogens you should inform your doctor who will monitor your blood thyroxine levels more closely and adjust your therapy accordingly.

How to eat more phytoestrogens

As we have seen, studies suggest that we need to eat at least 45 mg of phytoestrogens per day to have a beneficial effect. The richest dietary sources include soybeans and foods made from these, lentils, chickpeas, sprouting beans, linseeds, rye, most cereals, and fruit and vegetables. Reading this list it may strike you that the richest sources are foods that you never eat, for example soy and linseeds. Don't panic—you don't need to turn into a seed-nibbling vegetarian. There are many simple and easy ways to incorporate these into your daily diet. It is possible to achieve this without lots of home cooking, but the recipes in this book provide great ideas to add interest and variety to your diet.

Imitating nature
A synthetic phytoestrogen (Ipriflavone) is used to treat osteoporosis. The effective dose of this drug is, however, much, much higher than could be achieved by dietary means (200–600 mg per day, compared to the 50–100 mg in a traditional soy-rich Japanese diet).

How much do foods contain?

The phytoestrogen content of foods will vary, and processing may reduce a food's content. Many foods with phytoestrogen-rich ingredients, such as soy or linseeds, do not provide information on the label with the actual phytoestrogen content. Rather than trying to count phytoestrogens, therefore, the best approach is to become familiar with the foods that contain them and to aim to include these in your diet several times each day.

Should I take supplements?

In short, no. Despite the fact that millions of dollars are spent on phytoestrogen supplements around the world each year, studies have found that naturally-occurring phytoestrogens are far more effective than those presented as pills.

Reliability is also a problem. When phytoestrogen supplements have been analyzed, over two-thirds have been found to contain fewer phytoestrogens than the amount claimed by the manufacturer. As a result, experts advise women to consume their phytoestrogens as foods, not pills.

One simple solution

To get 45 mg of phytoestrogens, you need three servings of a phytoestrogen-rich food each day. Try the following simple solution:
1 Two slices of a soy or linseed bread
2 One serving of a phyto-rich granola
3 Use soy milk in your tea or coffee, or make a fruit smoothie with soy milk

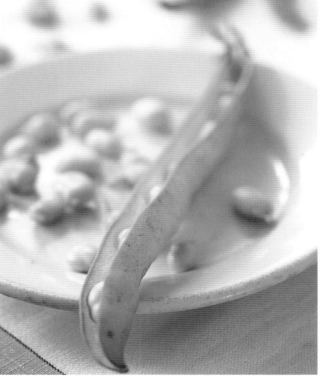

right All beans and legumes contain phytoestrogens.

Great phytoestrogen-rich choices

Food		Phytoestrogens per 3½ oz	Average serving	Phytoestrogens per serving
Textured vegetable protein (TVP)		75 mg	2½ oz	56 mg
Tofu		13.5–67 mg	3½ oz	40 mg
Linseeds (flaxseeds)		60–370 mg	1 tablespoon	31 mg
Banana & Mango Smoothie (see page 42)			8-oz glass	30 mg
Soybeans		37 mg	3 tablespoons	28 mg
Soy flour		131–198 mg	1 tablespoon	25 mg

Food		Phytoestrogens per 3½ oz	Average serving	Phytoestrogens per serving
Soy milk		5–10 mg	8-oz glass	12.5–25 mg
Strawberry Granola (see page 34)			1 bowl with ⅔ cup soy milk	20 mg
Miracle Bread (see page 132)			2 slices	12 mg
Tempeh		29–53 mg	1 oz	10 mg
Soy cheese		6–31 mg	1¾-oz slice	9 mg
Miso		45 mg	1 tablespoon	7 mg
Meat-free soy burgers		8–15 mg	1¾-oz burger	6 mg

Food		Phytoestrogens per 3½ oz	Average serving	Phytoestrogens per serving
Blackberries		4 mg	²/₃ cup	4 mg
Gooseberries		3 mg	²/₃ cup	3 mg
China green tea/black tea		3 mg/1.1 mg	1 cup	3 mg/1.1 mg
Peas		3.28 mg	1 cup	1.6 mg
Lentils		3.28 mg	½ cup	1.6 mg
Split peas		3.28 mg	¼ cup	1.6 mg
Chianti/Cabernet Sauvignon wine		1.1 mg	4-oz glass	1.4 mg
Dried currants and raisins		2 mg	⅓ cup (small handful)	1.0 mg
Brown rice		0.3 mg	½ cup	0.3 mg

Lifestyle approaches to menopause

There are a number of other changes you can make to reduce the severity of menopausal symptoms. These include:

- Avoiding getting too warm by dressing in layers so you can easily add and remove them in response to different room temperatures
- Sleeping in a cool room
- Keeping your temperature down by avoiding hot drinks and hot soups
- Avoiding triggers for hot flashes such as alcohol or spicy foods
- Developing effective ways of dealing with stress and learning to relax
- When a hot flash starts to develop, taking slow, deep breaths, which may lessen the severity
- Getting regular moderate exercise
- Maintaining a healthy body weight
- Having your blood pressure checked regularly
- If you have diabetes, ensuring that your blood sugar control is good

Nontraditional therapies

There are many alternative therapies that may help to alleviate some of the stress of menopause, including acupuncture, meditation, massage, and other relaxation techniques. Although no scientific evidence exists to suggest that these work, they will certainly not harm, and some women report great benefit from them. Some women also try herbal supplements such as Black Cohosh, Dong Quai, and Ginseng. Always talk to your doctor before embarking on any of these therapies.

below Remember to take time for yourself and to relax.

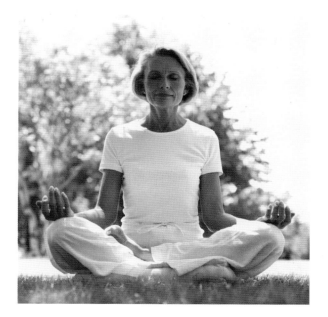

Heart disease and menopause

Increasing the risk

Other factors that increase your risk of heart disease include:

- smoking
- high blood pressure
- diabetes
- high blood cholesterol levels
- inactivity
- being overweight
- alcohol intake
- low intake of fruit and vegetables

below Oily fish are the richest source of omega 3 fatty acids. Try to eat some at least once a week.

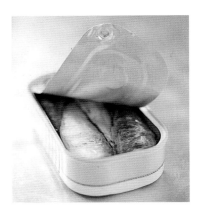

It is a common but mistaken belief that heart disease affects men more than women. Heart disease is in fact the most common cause of death among both women and men in Western societies. During 2001, 126,000 women died of heart disease in the UK—that's 50,000 more than cancer, so this cannot be overlooked as a serious health concern.

Heart disease occurs as a result of two processes, which develop gradually over many years. The first process, atherosclerosis, is a buildup of cholesterol in the outer walls of the blood vessels in the heart (similar to scale building up inside a pipe), which reduces blood flow. When the heart works harder during exertion or times of increased emotion, the amount of blood flowing may be too low to meet demand, resulting in pain (angina).

The second process, thrombosis, occurs if the cholesterol deposits crack, allowing a blood clot to form and block a blood vessel completely. This is what happens during a heart attack where the blood flow to part of the heart is cut off, resulting in permanent damage to that area of the heart.

Before menopause, women are protected against heart disease by the hormone estrogen. As menopause progresses and estrogen levels decline, the incidence of heart disease in women rapidly escalates and within a few years matches that of men.

Four steps to a healthy heart

1 Eat healthily Avoid eating too much saturated fat, eat plenty of fish, poultry, fruit, and vegetables and maintain a healthy body weight.

2 Be more active Half an hour every day is enough to make a difference and it's easy to build into your daily routine. Start off gently and gradually build up.

3 Quit smoking From the moment you stop smoking your risk of heart attack starts to fall and is halved within one year of giving up.

4 Reduce your alcohol intake Binge drinking increases your risk of having a heart attack.

What affects your heart?

Negative factors

Low intake of fruit and vegetables Currently less than one in three people eat at least five portions a day. If we all ate five a day, the incidence of heart disease, stroke, and cancers would fall by 20 percent.

Saturated fats These are mainly found in animal foods such as butter, cream, lard, fatty meats, burgers, and sausages but also in some vegetable sources, particularly palm oil and coconut. Choose lean cuts of meat and eat fewer processed meat products.

Adding extra fats Try to limit the amount of fat that you add to foods. Spread margarine or butter thinly, and eat tomato, rather than cream-based, sauces. Select your cooking method carefully. Stir-fry, boil, or casserole. Eat fried foods only rarely. Do not add fat when roasting meat.

Raised cholesterol levels Often caused by a diet high in saturated fats. If your cholesterol level is high, choose a cholesterol-lowering spread in place of butter or margarine.

Low-fiber diet This leaves you feeling hungry and constipated. Even slight constipation makes you feel sluggish and dull. Increasing fiber intake reduces fatigue and boosts energy levels by 10 percent.

Weight gain Bad for your self-esteem and your general health. The most common cause is inactivity, so get out there and be as active as you can, as often as you can.

Positive factors

Antioxidants These hugely beneficial chemicals found in fruit and vegetables come in a wide range of colors, so try to eat fruit and vegetables of all colors and at least five portions every day. Also found in red wine and grape juice.

Polyunsaturated and monounsaturated fats These help to moderate cholesterol levels if eaten in moderation. They include olive, sunflower, soy, canola, and corn oils, and spreads or margarines made from these. Always use fats in moderation.

Soy and phytoestrogens Phytoestrogen-rich soy foods are proven to lower cholesterol levels and protect the heart. Try to include three servings of a soy food in your diet daily.

Oily fish Try to eat herring, mackerel, trout, salmon, or sardines once or twice every week.

High-fiber cereal foods These provide a long-lasting source of energy, keep you feeling full, and offer a great source of dietary fiber, which helps to control cholesterol and blood sugar levels. Choose whole-grain breads and cereals and whole-wheat pasta as often as you can.

Increased activity This helps the heart and muscles get fitter and boosts the metabolism, helping with weight control. It is the best form of stress relief, helps control anxiety and depression, and is a fantastic mood-enhancer. If you want to feel and look great, get active.

Managing weight during menopause

Around the time of menopause, many women have problems maintaining their normal body weight. In fact, by the age of 55–64 years, three-quarters of women are overweight or obese. While there is no direct evidence that menopause is a cause of weight gain in itself, the symptoms of menopause may dampen your enthusiasm for exercise. Also, other lifestyle changes may be affecting both your eating and activity levels, such as your children leaving home or an increase of available cash because the mortgage has been paid off. It does not take much of an imbalance between energy intake and energy expenditure for the weight to suddenly start creeping up.

below Remember to drink plenty of fluids to stave off hunger and flush away toxins.

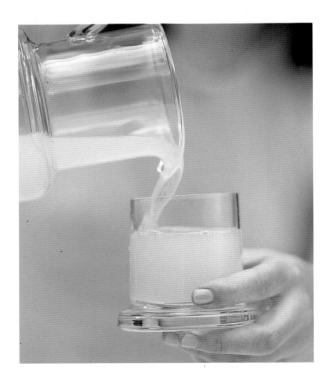

Why worry about your weight?

It is uncomfortable to be large, but a more pressing concern is the impact on your health. Carrying extra body fat places a strain on the heart, stresses the immune system, making you more susceptible to infections, makes you more likely to have joint problems, and increases the risk of diseases such as diabetes, cancer, gallstones, and heart disease. Important too is where you carry your weight. Weight around your middle is most damaging to health. For women, if your waist is bigger than 31½ inches, then now is the time to take action. For men, a waist measurement greater than 37 inches requires a change in lifestyle.

While "quick-fix" diets promising overnight weight loss are tempting, remember they are just that—a quick fix that is temporary. The most effective approach to long-term weight control is a combination of healthy eating and increased activity levels.

Keeping active

Inactivity is the main cause of gradual weight gain. Only one-quarter of women achieve the recommended activity levels of 30 minutes of moderate activity per day. Becoming more active should be a major focus for anyone trying to manage their weight. And we are not just talking about getting down to the gym. How many hours each day do you spend sitting down? Think about all the times through the day that you could be more active—whether it is finding time for a quick walk, washing the car by hand instead of driving to the car wash, going bowling rather than spending another evening in front of the television, or using the stairs instead of taking the elevator.

It is surprising how quickly lots of little bits of extra activity through a day can add up to make you more fit and keep you burning off the calories. If you simply found the time to have a 20-minute brisk walk every day for a year, then you could burn off 11 lb of body fat. Not a huge amount of effort, but the potential for great results.

above Being active with friends is easier than going alone.

Keeping a diary

We often don't realize how much or how often we eat each day, or how inactive we actually are. Keeping a food and activity diary can be the prompt we need to become more aware of our habits and to start to make changes to them. Try keeping a diary for a few days to become more aware of what you are doing at different times of day or in different situations.

Be as honest as possible in your diary and then take a critical look at your habits. Consider the following:

• Are you eating regular meals—do you include breakfast every day?
• Are you eating at least five portions of fruit and vegetables every day?
• How often do you eat and drink between meals?
• Are there any times when you could be more active?
• Are there times when you choose not to be active?

Food and activity dairy

Time of day	What food or what activity?	How much?	Who with?	How I felt
Breakfast	Bowl of cereal with skim milk and sugar 2 cups of tea	Medium bowl $\frac{1}{3}$ pint 2 teaspoons 2 cups	The family	Rushed at the start of the day
Midmorning	Cup of tea with a banana	1 cup 1 medium	Alone at my desk	Hungry
Lunch	Walking Sandwich made with reduced-fat cheese and tomatoes Cup of tea with milk	45 minutes 2 slices bread 2 slices cheese 5 cherry tomatoes 1 cup	A friend	Fabulous. Came back from the walk feeling hot but energized. Needed the sandwich and cup of tea afterward, but felt alert for the rest of the day.

Making changes

After taking a careful look at your habits, now is the time to start making some changes. Setting yourself goals is easy—but achieving them is hard. This is often because the goals that we set are not achievable or are simply the wrong goals. Goals should always be challenging enough to take us into new territory and to do things that we have not managed before—after all, what is the point of putting in all of the effort otherwise? However, we do need to make sure that they will give us the end results we want. Learning how to set goals that work takes practice and patience—we also need to learn from a few failures to get better at doing this.

Introduction **27**

The rules of SMART goals

Always make sure your goals include the following elements:

S—Specific What are you actually going to do? A specific goal would be to cut down the number of French fries you eat from three servings a week to just one. A nonspecific goal would be to "eat fewer French fries."

M—Measurable Always include numbers in your goals so you know if you are successful. For example, walk for 20 minutes twice each week—you can easily see if you are achieving this goal.

A—Achievable A goal has to be tough but achievable. If at the moment you never go out for a walk, setting a goal to walk every day for an hour is going to be tough! Set something more realistic, such as walking twice a week. Once you can do that, make it more challenging.

R—Realistic Don't be scared to set small goals in order to work up to reaching a bigger goal that at the moment feels impossible. What will achieving the goal give you? The toughest goals will give you the greatest boost, so be realistic about the work involved, commit to doing it, and then get going.

T—Time specific Set a timescale to review your goals every few weeks to see how you are doing.

If you don't meet your goals

We need to accept that sometimes we will not achieve what we set out to do. If this is the case, then resist the temptation to be negative. All too often we assume that we are a failure, weak-willed, and incapable of achieving success. There are many reasons why we fail to achieve—the trick is to use these occasions as a learning experience. Think about what you wanted to do. Was it SMART? How much of your goal did you manage to achieve and what went wrong? How could you do it differently next time?

Spend some time thinking about it rather than simply writing yourself off. Being able to set effective goals takes time and practice, and only by doing it will you become good at it. Above all, stick with it. The results are well worth achieving.

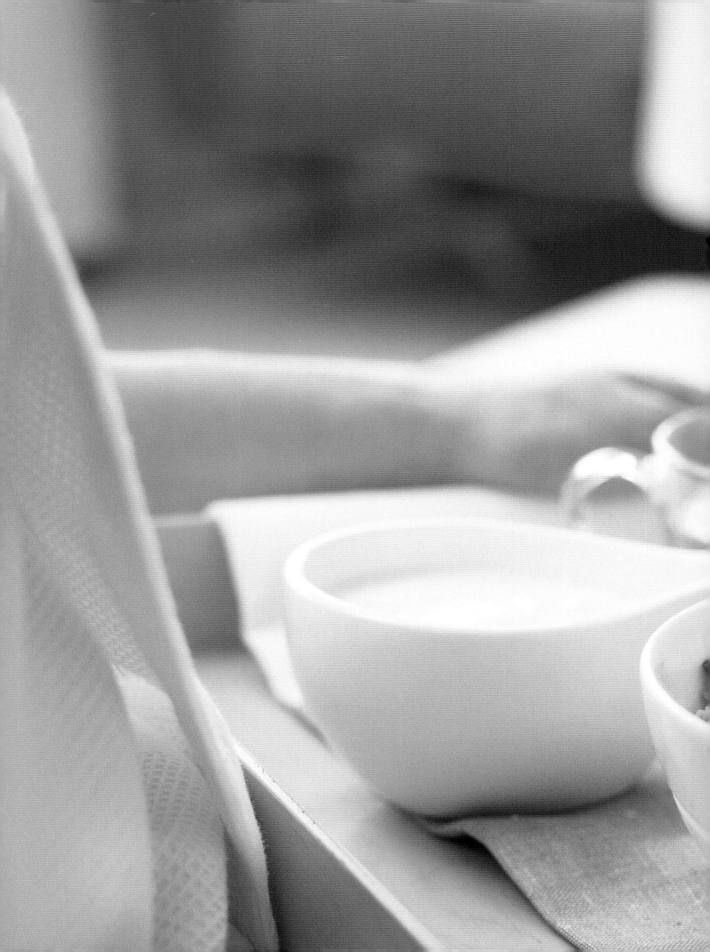

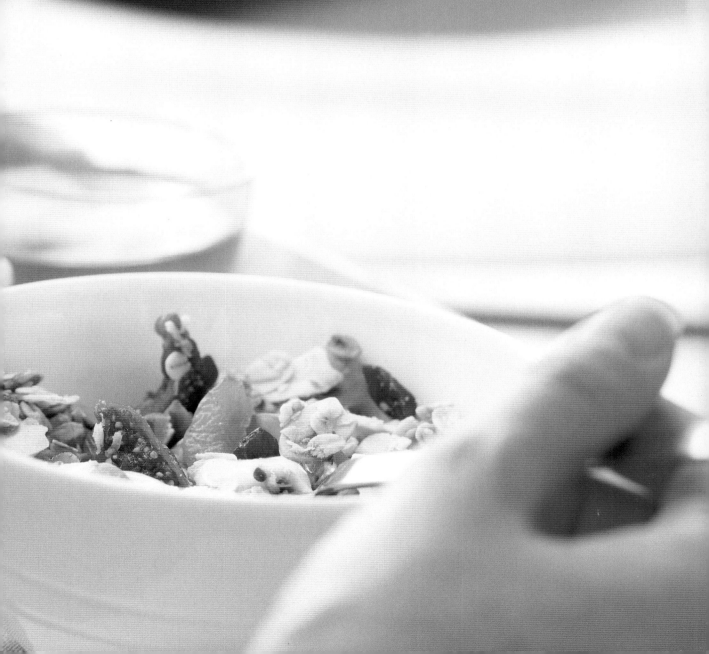

breakfasts

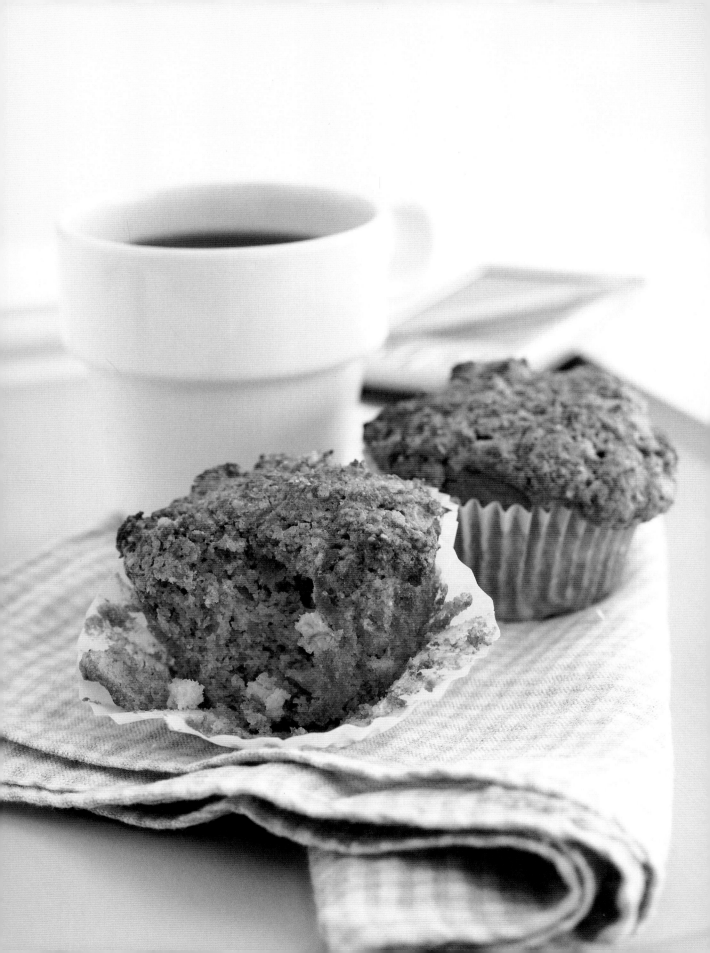

preparation time
15 minutes

cooking time
25–30 minutes

makes 6 muffins

nutritional values per muffin
- 250 kcals
- 10 g fat
- 2.5 g saturated fat
- 2.5 g fiber
- Source of phytoestrogens

Cook's tip
These muffins are best eaten fresh, but they will keep for 2–3 days in an airtight container.

banana muffins with cinnamon topping

butter, for greasing (optional)
3/ċ cup (100 g) whole-wheat flour
1/3 cup (25 g) soy flour
3 tablespoons light Barbados sugar
2 teaspoons baking powder
1 egg, beaten
1/4 cup (50 ml) soya milk
1/4 cup (50 ml) sunflower oil
1 cup (200 g) roughly mashed ripe bananas

Topping
1 tablespoon golden linseeds
1/4 cup (25 g) self-rising flour, sifted
1 tbsp (15 g) butter, at room temperature
1/3 cup (40 g) Demerara sugar
1/2 teaspoon ground cinnamon
1 tablespoon water

As well as making a delicious breakfast, these tasty muffins make a great portable snack for when you are on the move.

1 Line 6 muffin cups with paper bake cups or grease the cups well. Begin by making the topping. Place the linseeds in a blender or food processor and process for 30 seconds. Alternatively, grind them in a clean coffee grinder. Place the self-rising flour in a bowl and cut in the butter until the mixture resembles fine breadcrumbs. Add the sugar, linseeds, and cinnamon, then stir in the measured water and mix well.

2 Place the whole-wheat and soy flours, sugar, and baking powder in a bowl, mix together and make a well in the center. In a separate bowl, mix the egg, soy milk, and oil together. Pour the liquid into the flour. Stir until just blended. Stir in the mashed banana, being careful not to overmix.

3 Fill the muffin cups two-thirds full with the mixture, then sprinkle a little of the topping over each muffin. Place in a preheated oven at 400°F for 20–35 minutes or until a skewer inserted into the center comes out clean. Transfer the muffins to a wire rack to cool.

preparation time
10 minutes

cooking time
5 minutes

makes 10–12 servings

nutritional values per serving
- 364–304 kcals
- 26–17 g fat
- 10–6 g saturated fat
- 6–4 g fiber
- Source of phytoestrogens

Cook's tip
The granola can be stored in an airtight container for up to 1 month.

granola

¹/₃ cup (75 g) butter
¹/₃ cup honey
1 teaspoon vanilla extract
2¹/₂ cups (300 g) regular rolled oats
²/₃ cup (50 g) dried shredded coconut
¹/₂ cup (50 g) sliced almonds
3 tablespoons sunflower seeds
3 tablespoons pumpkin seeds
1 tablespoon sesame seeds
1 tablespoon linseeds
3 oz (75 g) rye flakes
3 oz (75 g) mixed dried fruit, roughly chopped

1 Place the butter, honey, and vanilla extract in a small saucepan. Cook over a medium heat, stirring occasionally, for 5 minutes or until the honey and butter are combined.

2 Place all the remaining ingredients, except the fruit, in a large bowl and mix well. Carefully stir in the butter mixture. Spread the mixture over the base of a large, nonstick baking sheet and place in a preheated oven at 325°F for 20 minutes or until the grains are crisp and browned. Stir occasionally to prevent the mixture from sticking.

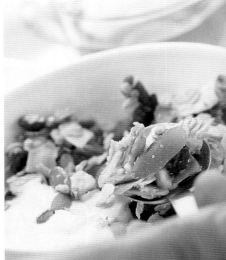

3 Remove from the oven and allow to cool. Stir in the dried fruit.

preparation time
5 minutes

cooking time
5–10 minutes

serves 2

nutritional values per serving
- 255 kcals
- 4 g fat
- 0.5 g saturated fat
- 3 g fiber
- Source of phytoestrogens

Cook's tip
Instead of bananas try
adding a handful of fresh
berries or a few roughly
chopped dried apricots.

banana porridge

1 cup (75 g) regular rolled oats
1/2 cup (100 ml) soy milk
1/3 cup (75 ml) water
1 tablespoon brown sugar
1/2 cup (125 g) finely sliced ripe banana
To serve
extra soy milk
pumpkin seeds

1 Place the oats, soy milk, water, sugar, and banana in a heavy saucepan. Bring to a boil, stirring steadily. Reduce the heat and simmer, stirring occasionally, for 5–10 minutes, or until the desired consistency is reached.

2 Spoon into bowls. Pour a little more soy milk over each portion and scatter a few pumpkin seeds on top.

preparation time
5 minutes

cooking time
2–2¹/2 hours

makes 12–14 servings

nutritional values per serving
- 229–200 kcals
- 12–10 g fat
- 1–0.7 g saturated fat
- 3–2.5 g fiber
- Source of phytoestrogens

Cook's tip
The granola can be stored for up to about 3 weeks in an airtight container.

strawberry granola

1¹/3 cups (250 g) strawberries, thinly sliced
3 cups (250 g) regular rolled oats
³/4 cup (75 g) sliced almonds
¹/2 cup (75 g) pumpkin seeds
¹/2 cup (75 g) sunflower seeds
2 tbsp (25 g) golden linseeds
¹/2 cup (75 g) dried cranberries, roughly chopped
soy milk, to serve

1 Blot away any juice from the strawberries with paper towels and set them in a single layer on a baking sheet lined with parchment paper. Place in a preheated oven at 225°F for 1 hour. Turn them over and continue to bake for a further 1–1¹/2 hours, or until crisp. Allow to cool.

2 Mix together the remaining ingredients, carefully stir in the strawberries, and store the mixture in an airtight container. When ready to serve, pour into bowls and add a splash of soy milk.

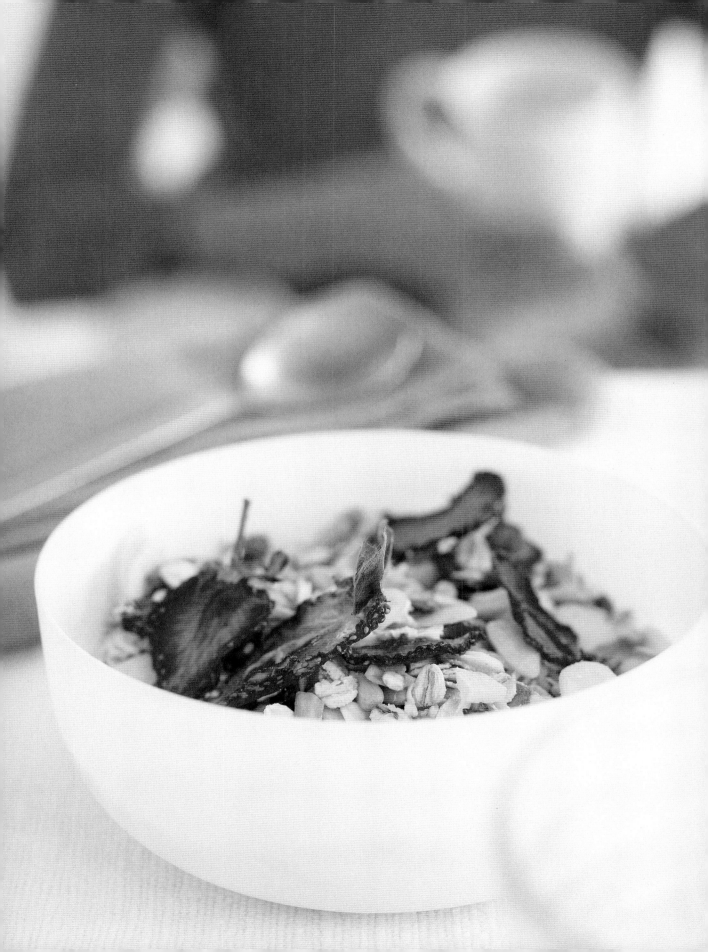

preparation time
5 minutes

serves 2

nutritional values per serving
- 300 kcals
- 11 g fat
- 1.5 g saturated fat
- 3 g fiber
- Source of phytoestrogens

lemon and passionfruit yogurt with granola

2 tablespoons lemon curd
4 tablespoons Strawberry Granola (see page 34), or other sugar-free granola
1¾ cups (400 ml) plain soy yogurt
3 passionfruit

1 Stir the lemon curd and the granola into the soy yogurt and spoon the mixture into 2 dishes. Remove the seeds and pulp from the passionfruit and drizzle over the yogurt. Serve immediately.

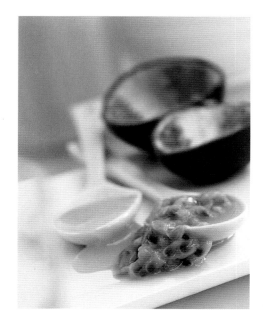

preparation time
10 minutes

cooking time
15 minutes

serves 2

nutritional values per serving
- 230 kcals
- 9 g fat
- 1 g saturated fat
- 2 g fiber
- Source of phytoestrogens

spiced apricots with yogurt

$2/3$ cup (75 g) dried apricots, roughly chopped
$2/3$ cup (150 ml) unsweetened orange juice
1 cardamom pod, seeds removed and lightly crushed
$1^2/3$ cups (400 ml) plain soy yogurt

1 Place the apricots, orange juice, and crushed cardamom seeds in a small saucepan and gently heat. As soon as the orange juice begins to boil, reduce the heat, cover, and simmer for 10 minutes.

2 Transfer the apricot mixture to a blender or food processor and puree until smooth, adding a little more juice if necessary. Allow the mixture to cool.

3 Stir the apricot puree into the soy yogurt and serve.

preparation time
5 minutes

cooking time
4–8 minutes

serves 2

nutritional values per serving
- 234 kcals
- 10 g fat
- 5 g saturated fat
- 2 g fiber
- Source of phytoestrogens

Cook's tip
If you like, try using Burgen bread for this recipe—it is also high in phytoestrogens.

pain perdu with fruit compote

2 slices Miracle Bread (see page 132)
1 egg, beaten
3 tablespoons soy milk
1 drop vanilla extract, or a pinch of ground cinnamon
1 tbsp (15 g) butter
2 tablespoons light brown sugar
Summer Fruit Compote (see page 120), to serve

1 Cut the slices of bread in half diagonally. Beat together the egg, milk, and vanilla or cinnamon. Heat the butter in a nonstick skillet. Dip the bread slices in the egg mixture until well coated.

2 When the butter is foaming, add the bread and sprinkle over half the sugar. Cook over a medium heat for 2–3 minutes. Turn over, sprinkle with the remaining sugar, and cook for a further 2 minutes.

3 Serve immediately with the fruit compote.

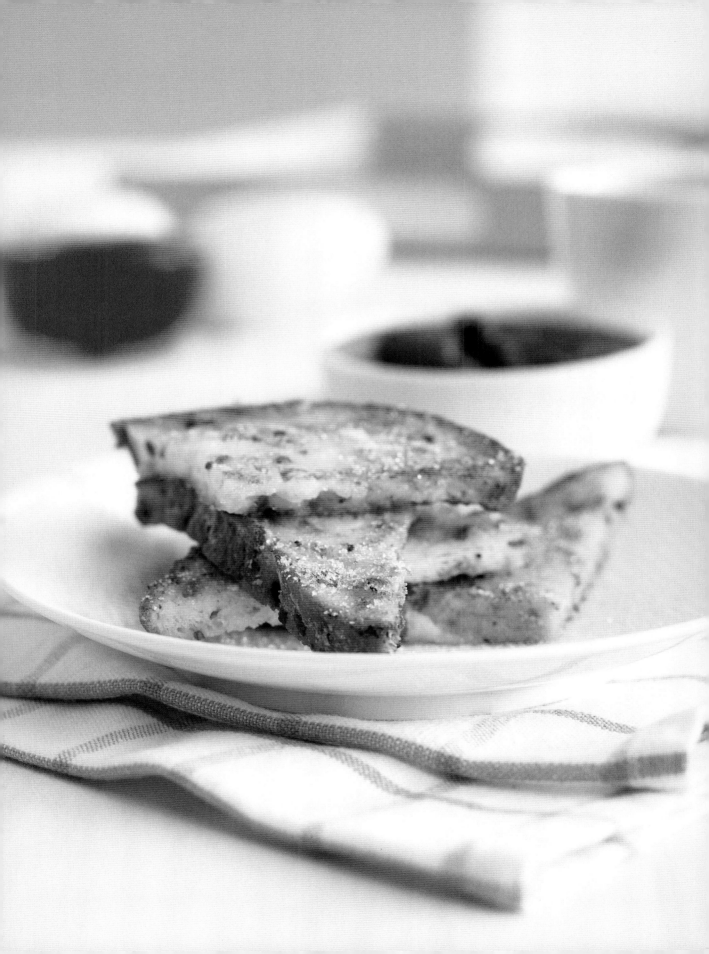

preparation time
5 minutes

cooking time
2–3 minutes

serves 2

nutritional values per serving
- 211 kcals
- 12 g fat
- 5 g saturated fat
- 0 g fiber
- Good source of phytoestrogens

spiced chocolate milk

500 ml (17 fl oz) soy milk
2 oz (50 g) unsweetened or semisweet
chocolate, grated
1 teaspoon honey
¼ teaspoon ground cardamom

1 Place the soy milk in a small saucepan and heat gently. Whisk in the remaining ingredients, then pour into mugs and serve immediately.

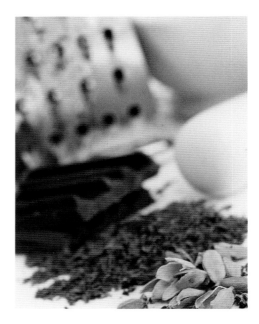

preparation time
5 minutes

cooking time
10 minutes

serves 2

nutritional values per serving
- 50 kcals
- 3 g fat
- 0.5 g saturated fat
- 0 g fiber
- Good source of phytoestrogens

Cook's tip
Fresh soy milk has a much better flavor than soy milk sold in long-life cartons.

almond soy latte

1¼ cups (300 ml) soy milk
4 drops of almond extract
2/3 cup (150 ml) hot espresso coffee
sugar, to taste

1 Place the soy milk in a saucepan and slowly bring to a boil, stirring occasionally. Pour the milk into two tall, heatproof glasses.

2 Add the almond extract to the coffee, then stir into the milk. Add sugar to taste and serve.

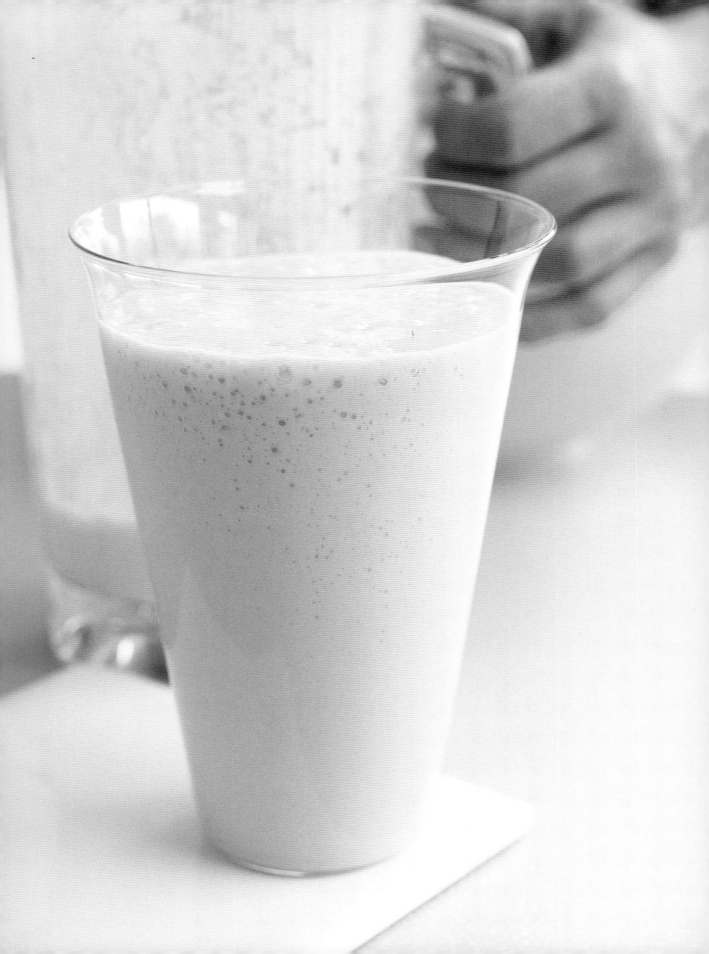

preparation time
2 minutes, plus freezing

serves 1

nutritional values per serving
- 230 kcals
- 3 g fat
- 0.5 g saturated fat
- 2 g fiber
- Good source of phytoestrogens

banana and mango smoothie

1 small ripe banana, about
3¹/₂ oz (100 g)
1 cup (250 ml) soy milk
1 small ripe mango, seeded, peeled,
and diced

1 Peel and slice the banana, then place in a freezerproof container and freeze for at least 2 hours or overnight.

2 Place all the ingredients in a blender or food processor and blend until thick and frothy. Pour into a glass and serve immediately.

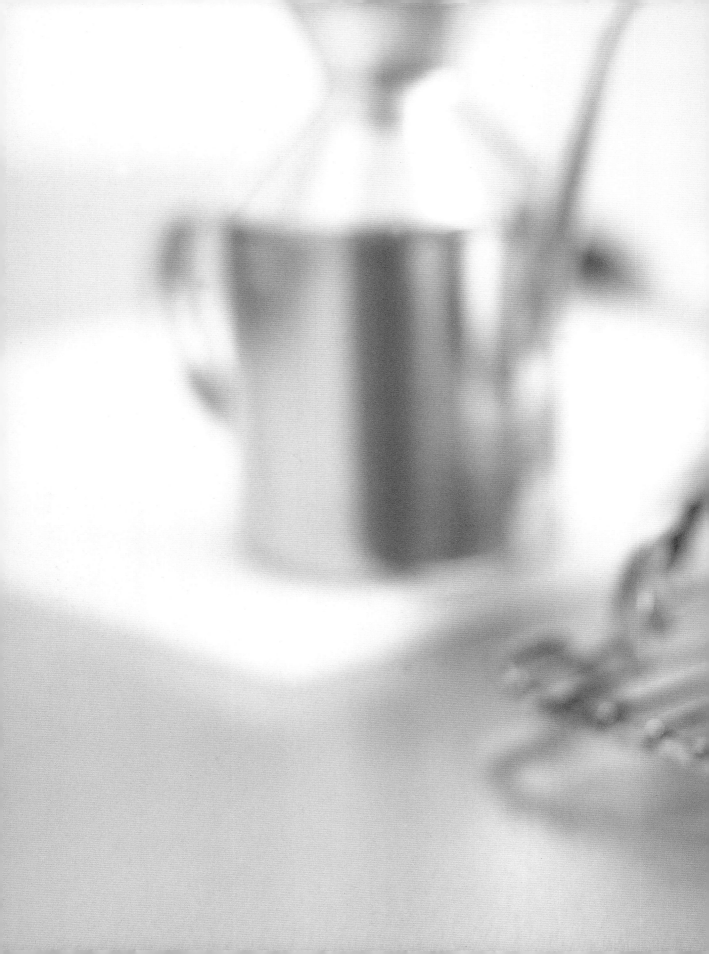

light bites

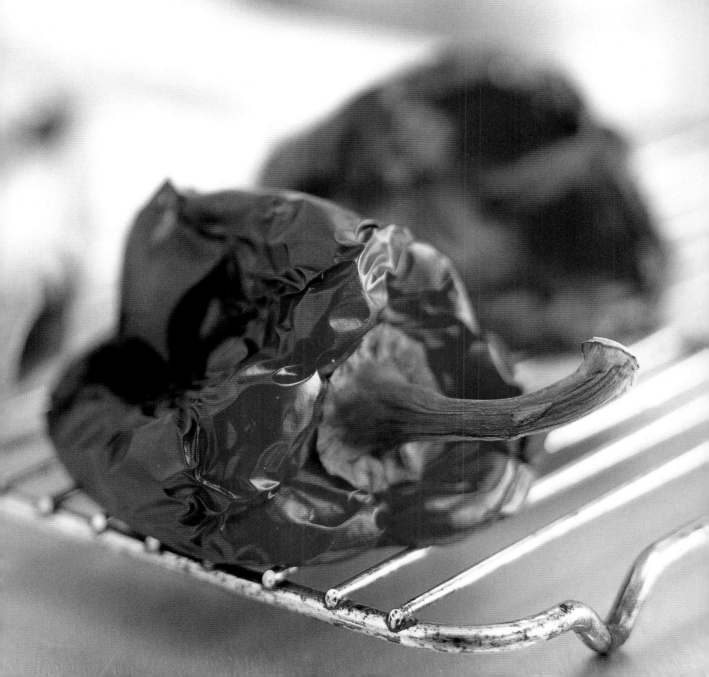

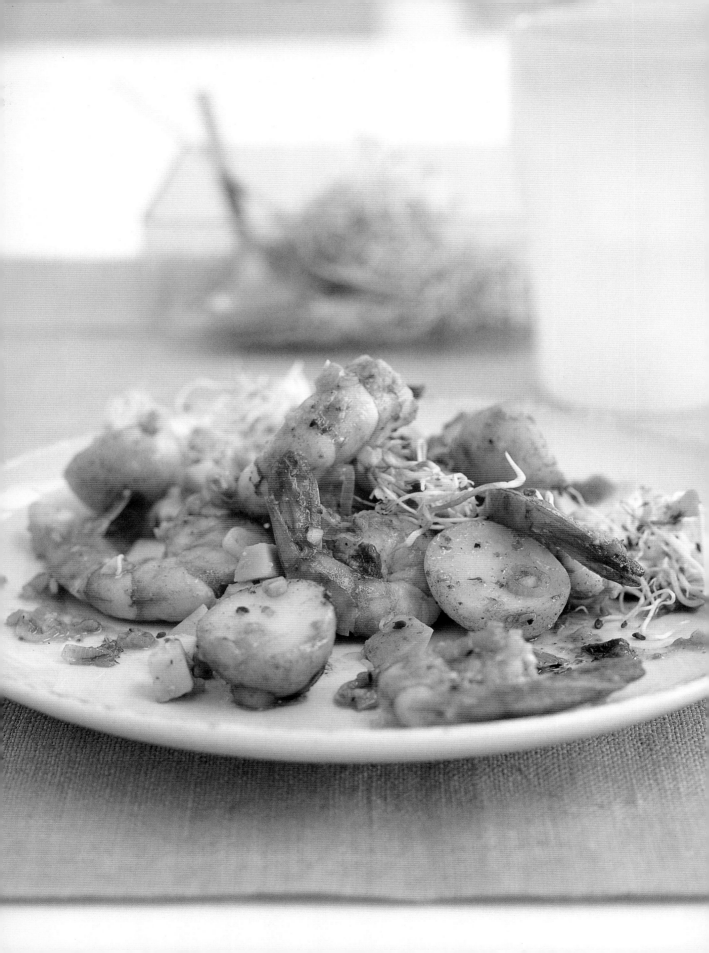

preparation time
10 minutes

cooking time
10–15 minutes

serves 2

nutritional values per serving
- 440 kcals
- 23 g fat
- 4.5 g saturated fat
- 4.5 g fiber

Cook's tip
Give the potatoes a good wash but leave the skins on to increase the fiber content.

cajun potato, shrimp, and avocado salad

10 oz (300 g) baby new potatoes, scrubbed and halved
1 tablespoon olive oil
8 oz (250 g) cooked peeled jumbo shrimp
I garlic clove, crushed
4 green onions, finely sliced
2 teaspoons Cajun seasoning
1 ripe avocado, peeled, seeded, and diced
handful of alfalfa sprouts
salt

1 Cook the potatoes in a large saucepan of lightly salted boiling water for 10–15 minutes, or until tender. Drain well.

2 Heat the oil in a wok or large, nonstick skillet. Add the shrimp, garlic, green onions, and Cajun seasoning, and sauté for 2–3 minutes, or until the shrimp are hot. Stir in the potatoes and cook for a further 1 minute. Transfer to a serving dish.

3 Stir in the avocado, top with the alfalfa sprouts, and serve.

nutritional values per serving
- 320 kcals
- 29 g fat
- 5 g saturated fat
- 5 g fiber
- Source of phytoestrogens

green salad with toasted mixed seeds

1 tablespoon sunflower seeds
1 tablespoon pumpkin seeds
2 teaspoons sesame seeds
2 teaspoons golden linseeds
pinch of driedchili flakes
2 tablespoons dark soy sauce
1³/₄ cups (50 g) mixed baby salad leaves
1/2 small cucumber, sliced
2 green onions, finely chopped
1 small avocado, peeled, seeded, and diced
Miracle Bread (see page 132), to serve

1 Place the seeds, dried chili flakes, and soy sauce in a bowl and mix well. Heat a small, heavy skillet, add the seed mixture, and cook for 5 minutes, stirring continuously.

2 Mix the remaining ingredients together in a serving bowl, sprinkle with the seed mixture, and serve with Miracle Bread.

preparation time
10 minutes

cooking time
10–15 minutes

serves 2

nutritional values per serving
- 250 kcals
- 14 g fat
- 1 g saturated fat
- 8 g fiber
- Source of phytoestrogens

tuna and flageolet bean salad

10-oz (300-g) can or bottle of flageolet beans, drained and rinsed
4 ripe tomatoes, quartered
4 green onions, finely chopped
6-oz (185-g) can tuna (water-pack), drained and flaked
12 pitted black olives, roughly chopped
handful of flat-leaf parsley, roughly chopped
handful of arugula leaves
Miracle Bread (see page 132), to serve

Dressing
2 tablespoons extra virgin olive oil
1 tablespoon white wine vinegar
dash of mustard powder
dash of sugar
1/4 teaspoon crushed garlic
salt and freshly ground black pepper

1 Place the beans, tomatoes, green onions, tuna, olives, parsley, and arugula in a serving bowl and toss together.

2 Place all the dressing ingredients in a jar with a screw-top lid and shake vigorously to dissolve the sugar. Add the dressing to the salad and toss well to coat. Serve with Miracle Bread.

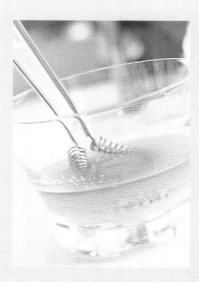

preparation time
10 minutes

cooking time
5 minutes

serves 2

nutritional values per serving
- 350 kcals
- 15 g fat
- 3 g saturated fat
- 8 g fiber
- Source of phytoestrogens

smoked chicken salad

10 5–7-inch long asparagus (about 160 g), cut into 2-inch (5-cm) lengths
7 oz (200 g) smoked chicken breast, cut into bite-sized pieces
8 cherry tomatoes (about 125 g), halved
1¼ cups (about 300 g) canned cannellini beans, drained and rinsed
handful of chives, chopped

Dressing
2 tablespoons olive oil
1 garlic clove, crushed
2 teaspoons honey
2 teaspoons balsamic vinegar
2 teaspoons prepared whole-grain mustard

1 Cook the asparagus in a large saucepan of lightly salted boiling water for about 4 minutes, or until just tender. Drain and plunge into cold water to prevent the asparagus from cooking further. Pat dry with kitchen towels.

2 Place the chicken in a large bowl, add the tomatoes, beans, asparagus, and chives and mix well.

3 To make the dressing, whisk all the ingredients together in a small bowl. Pour the dressing over the salad and toss well to coat.

Variation

If you can't find smoked chicken, use ordinary cooked chicken breast and chargrill the asparagus to add more flavor. Cook the asparagus in a large saucepan of lightly salted boiling water for 2–3 minutes. Drain well and pat dry with kitchen towels. Toss the asparagus with 1 tablespoon of olive oil and place on a hot griddle for 2–3 minutes, turning once, or until charred. Continue with Step 2 of the main recipe.

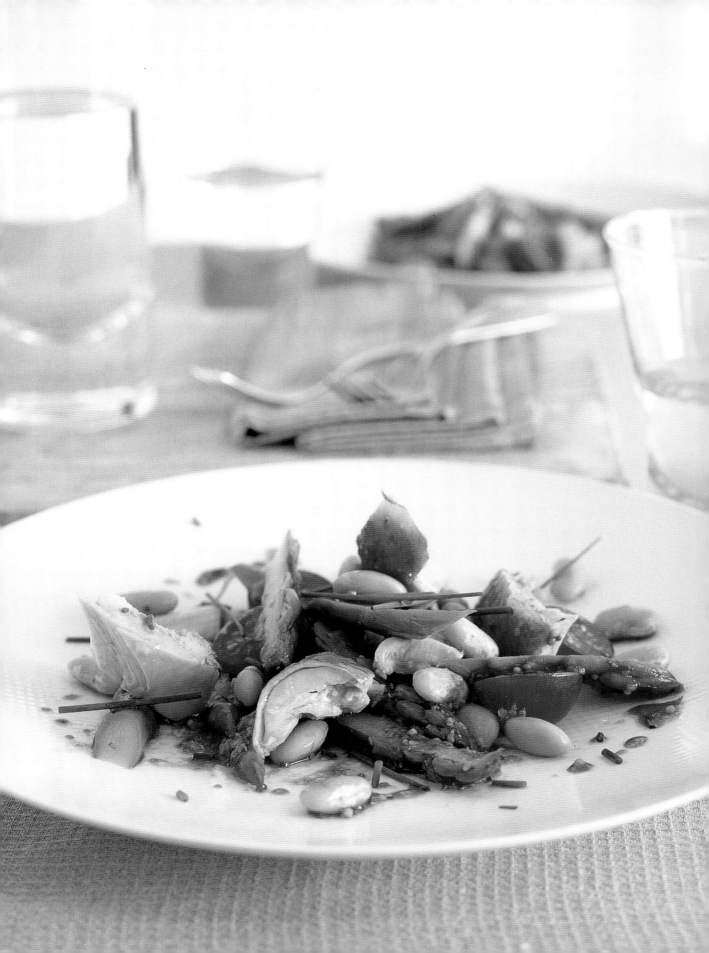

preparation time
10 minutes

cooking time
6–10 minutes

serves 2

nutritional values per serving
- 524 kcals
- 16 g fat
- 2 g saturated fat
- 10 g fiber
- Source of phytoestrogens

falafel with salad and pita breads

1³/₄ cups (400 g) canned chickpeas, drained and rinsed
1 garlic clove, crushed
2 tablespoons chopped fresh cilantro
1 small red onion, roughly chopped
¹/₂ teaspoon ground cumin
¹/₂ teaspoon ground turmeric
1 tablespoon tahini
¹/₂ teaspoon salt
¹/₂ cup (25 g) fresh white breadcrumbs
2 tablespoons water
all-purpose flour, for shaping
vegetable oil, for frying
To serve
2 whole-wheat pita breads, toasted
mixed salad greens
Tofu and Garlic Dip (see page 56)

1 Place the chickpeas, garlic, cilantro, onion, spices, tahini, salt, and breadcrumbs in a blender or food processor and process until finely chopped. Turn the mixture into a large bowl and add the measured water. Knead the mixture with your hands until it binds together, adding a little more water if necessary.

2 With floured hands, shape the mixture into 6 small patties. Heat 1 inch (2.5 cm) of vegetable oil in a large, deep skillet and fry the patties in batches for 2–3 minutes on each side. Drain on paper towels.

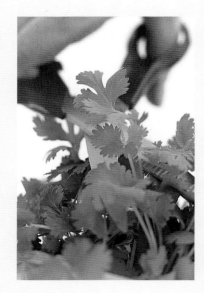

3 To serve, split open the toasted pita breads to make pockets. Fill with the falafel, plenty of mixed salad greens, and a tablespoon of Tofu and Garlic Dip.

preparation time
10 minutes

cooking time
10 minutes

serves 2

nutritional values per serving
- 265 kcals
- 10 g fat
- 1.5 g saturated fat
- 8 g fiber
- Source of phytoestrogens

Cook's tip
To skin tomatoes, place in a heatproof bowl, cover with boiling water, and leave to stand for 1 minute. Plunge the tomatoes into a bowl of ice-cold water. Peel off the skins.

spiced chickpea salad

1 tablespoon olive oil
1 red onion, finely chopped
1 teaspoon ground turmeric
2 teaspoons cumin seeds
2 medium tomatoes (about 300 g), skinned and roughly chopped
1 3/4 cups (400 g) canned chickpeas, drained and rinsed
2 teaspoons lemon juice
2 tablespoons chopped fresh cilantro
salt and freshly ground black pepper
Miracle Bread (see page 132), to serve

1 Heat the oil in a heavy skillet, add the onion, and sauté for 5 minutes, or until softened.

2 Add the turmeric and cumin seeds and cook, stirring, for 1–2 minutes. Add the tomatoes, chickpeas, lemon juice, and seasoning and cook for a further 2–3 minutes.

3 Stir in the chopped cilantro and serve with Miracle Bread.

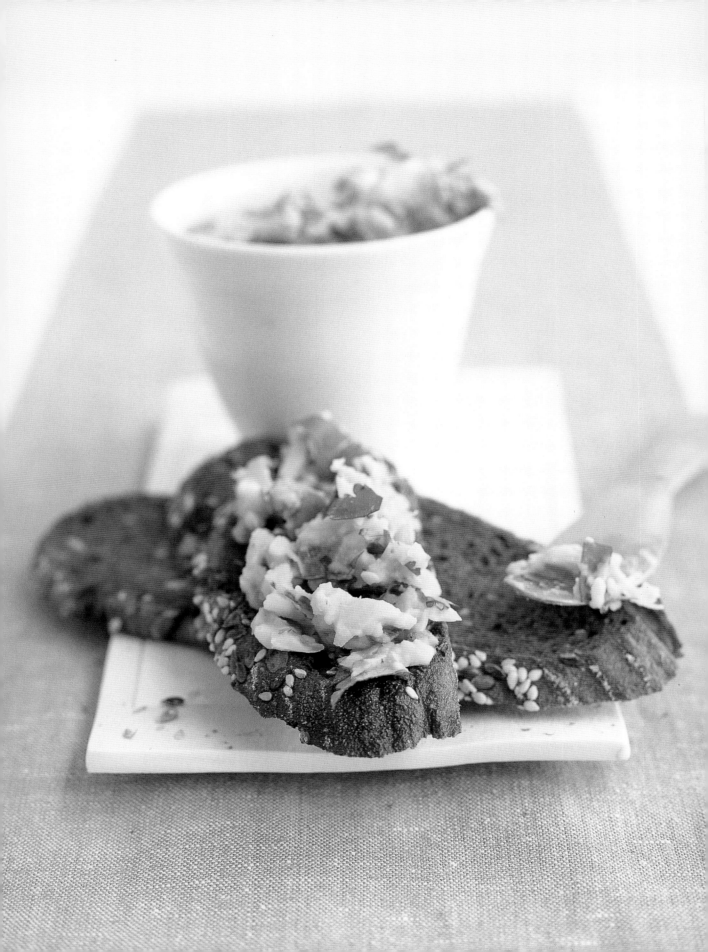

preparation time
5 minutes

serves 2–3

nutritional values per serving
- 260–170 kcals
- 11–7 g fat
- 1–0.5 g saturated fat
- 8–5.5 g fiber
- Source of phytoestrogens

Cook's tip
You can use other canned beans, such as cannellini or red kidney beans, in place of the Lima beans.

Lima bean, anchovy, and cilantro pâté

2¹/₃ cups (425 g) canned large Lima beans, drained and rinsed
12 anchovy fillets (about 50 g) canned in oil
2 green onions, finely chopped
2 tablespoons lemon juice
1 tablespoon olive oil
4 tablespoons chopped fresh cilantro
salt and freshly ground black pepper
To serve
lemon wedges
toasted rye bread

Serve this flavorsome pâté on toasted rye bread or Miracle Bread (see page 132).

1 Place all the ingredients, except the cilantro, in a blender or food processor. Puree until well mixed but not smooth. Alternatively, mash the beans with a fork, finely chop the anchovies, and mix the ingredients together by hand.

2 Stir in the cilantro and season well. Serve with lemon wedges and toasted rye bread.

preparation time
5 minutes

serves 4

nutritional values per serving
- 111 kcals
- 9 g fat
- 1 g saturated fat
- 0 g fiber
- Good source of phytoestrogens

tofu and garlic dip

11 oz (325 g) silken tofu
2 tablespoons extra virgin olive oil
2 large garlic cloves, crushed
1 teaspoon Dijon-style mustard
1^1/$_2$ tablespoons lemon juice
freshly ground black pepper

To serve
breadsticks
crudités

Serve this smooth, tangy dip with breadsticks and/or vegetable crudités, such as carrot, cucumber, red sweet pepper, and celery.

1 Place all the ingredients in a blender or food processor and puree until smooth. Season well with freshly ground black pepper.

2 Cover and chill until ready to serve. Serve with breadsticks and crudités.

preparation time
5 minutes

cooking time
15 minutes, plus cooling

serves 2

nutritional values per serving
- 180 kcals
- 14 g fat
- 2 g saturated fat
- 2 g fiber
- Good source of phytoestrogens

spicy red sweet pepper dip

1 large red sweet pepper (about 150 g)
5 oz (150 g) silken tofu
2 tablespoons olive oil
1 tablespoon sweet chili sauce
4 tablespoons hot water
salt and freshly ground black pepper
crudités, such as carrot and cucumber, to serve

1 Slice the sweet pepper in half and place, cut-side down, under a preheated hot broiler or skin-side down on a grill until the skin is blackened and the flesh soft. Place the pepper halves in a plastic bag and allow to cool for 15 minutes.

2 Skin the sweet peppers and remove the seeds and membrane. Then place the flesh in a blender or food processor with the tofu, oil, and chili sauce. Blend for 1 minute, then add the measured water and puree until smooth. Season well with salt and pepper.

3 Cover and chill for at least 2 hours to allow the flavors to develop. Taste and adjust the seasoning if necessary, then serve with crudités.

preparation time
15 minutes

cooking time
10 minutes

serves 2

nutritional values per serving
- 300 kcals
- 14 g fat
- 7 g saturated fat
- 8 g fiber
- Source of phytoestrogens

Cook's tip
To make crème fraîche combine 3 tbsp low-fat whipping cream (not ultra-pasteurized) and 3 tbsp low-fat dairy sour cream. Leave to stand at room temperature until it thickens (2–5 hours).

seared scallops with minted bean puree

1 tbsp (15 g) butter
2 shallots or 1/2 small onion, finely chopped
11/4 cups (about 300 g) canned fava beans, drained, rinsed, and outer shells removed
1 teaspoon mint sauce
6 tablespoons low-fat crème fraîche (see tip)
10 large scallops, shelled and cleaned
1 tablespoon olive oil
extra virgin olive oil, to drizzle
salt and freshly ground black pepper
mint sprigs, to garnish

1 Melt the butter in small saucepan and cook the shallots or onion over a medium heat for 5 minutes, or until softened. Place the shallots, beans, mint sauce, and crème fraîche in a blender or food processor and blend to make a coarse puree. Season to taste, then place in a clean saucepan and gently heat.

2 Brush the scallops with the olive oil, place on a hot griddle, and sear for 2 minutes on each side, or until browned and cooked through.

3 To serve, spoon a mound of bean puree onto 2 large white plates, and arrange 5 scallops around the edge of each plate. Drizzle with the extra virgin olive oil and garnish with mint sprigs and a grinding of black pepper.

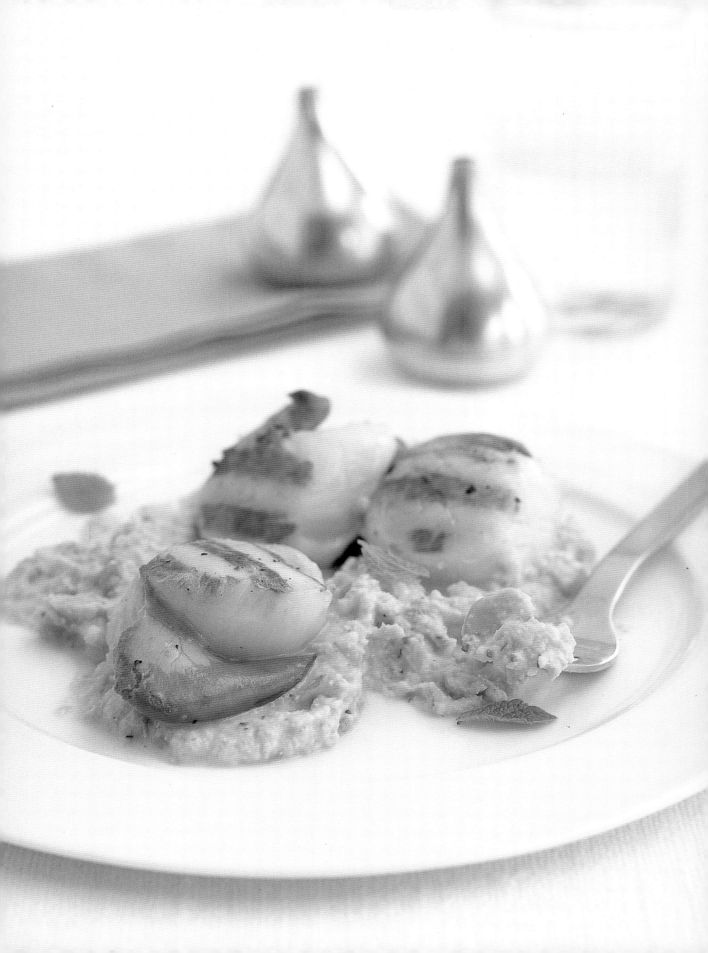

preparation time	nutritional values per serving
10 minutes	● 350 kcals
	● 20 g fat
cooking time	● 3 g saturated fat
5 minutes	● 8 g fiber
	● Source of phytoestrogens
serves 2	

hummus with dukkha

1³/4 cups (400 g) canned chickpeas, drained and rinsed

1 tablespoon tahini

2 tablespoons olive oil

2 garlic cloves, crushed

4 tablespoons lemon juice

3 tablespoons hot water

whole-wheat pita bread, toasted, to serve

Dukkha

2 tablespoons sesame seeds

1 tablespoon cumin seeds

¹/2 tablespoon ground coriander

¹/4 cup (25 g) hazelnuts (filberts), finely chopped

¹/4 teaspoon salt

Dukkha is an Egyptian spice mix made from a blend of nuts and seeds. It can be scattered over salads, used to top fish, or served as a nibble with a small dish of extra virgin olive oil and hot bread.

1 To make the pâté, place the chickpeas, tahini, oil, garlic, lemon juice, and measured water in a blender or food processor and process until smooth. Alternatively, mash the ingredients together with a fork.

2 To make the dukkha, toast the sesame and cumin seeds and coriander in a dry skillet over a low heat for 3 minutes, moving them around until they start to smell fragrant. Tip them out onto a plate. Add the hazelnuts to the skillet and sauté for 1–2 minutes, or until lightly golden. Stir the nuts and salt into the seed mixture. Store in an airtight container for up to 1 week.

3 Spread the pâté on whole-wheat pita bread and sprinkle with a little of the dukkha.

preparation time
15 minutes

cooking time
25 minutes

serves 2

nutritional values per serving
- 280 kcals
- 7 g fat
- 1 g saturated fat
- 11 g fiber
- Source of phytoestrogens

boston baked beans

1 tablespoon vegetable oil
1 small red onion, finely chopped
2 celery stalks, finely chopped
1 garlic clove, crushed
3/4 cup (200 g) canned chopped tomatoes
2/3 cup (150 ml) vegetable stock
1 tablespoon dark soy sauce
1 tablespoon dark brown sugar
2 teaspoons Dijon-style mustard
1 1/2 cups (400 g) canned mixed beans, drained and rinsed
2 tablespoons chopped parsley

Real homemade baked beans are a revelation. Serve on toasted seed bread for a light meal, or use as an accompaniment to sausages or grilled meat.

1 Heat the oil in heavy saucepan. Add the onion and cook over a low heat for 5 minutes, or until softened. Add the celery and garlic and continue to cook for 1–2 minutes.

2 Add the tomatoes, stock, and soy sauce. Bring to a boil, then reduce to a fast simmer and cook for about 15 minutes, or until the sauce begins to thicken.

3 Add the sugar, mustard, and beans. Continue to cook for a further 5 minutes, or until the beans are heated through. Stir in the chopped parsley and serve.

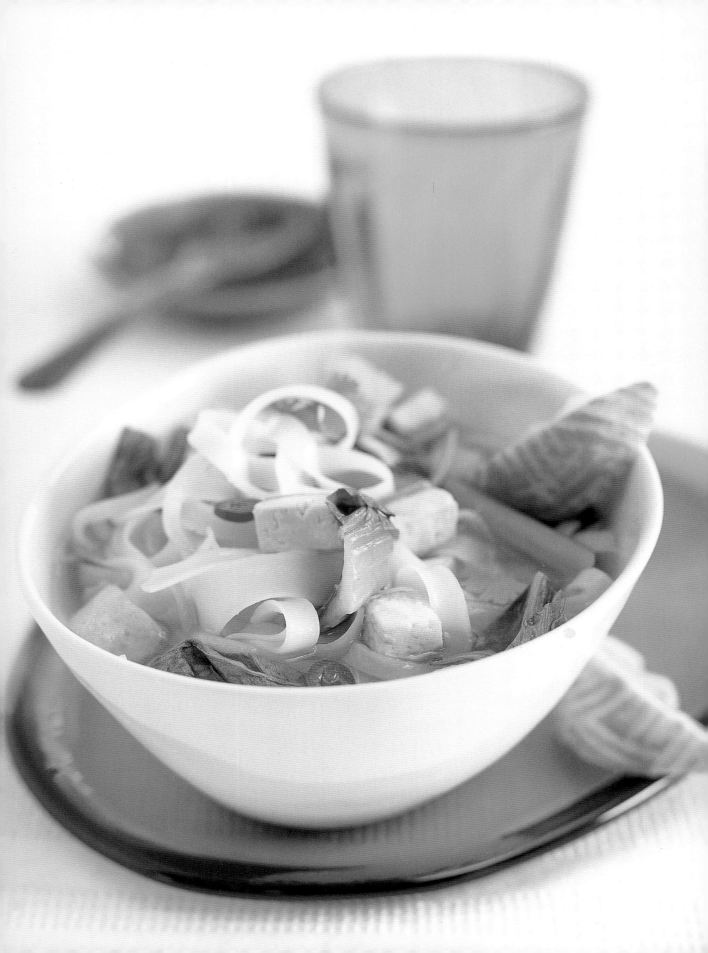

preparation time
10 minutes, plus draining

cooking time
10 minutes

serves 2

nutritional values per serving
- 250 kcals
- 8 g fat
- 1 g saturated fat
- 0.5 g fiber
- Good source of phytoestrogens

fragrant tofu and noodle soup

4 oz (125 g) firm tofu, diced
1 tablespoon sesame oil
3 oz (75 g) thin rice noodles
2 1/2 cups (600 ml) vegetable stock
1-inch (2.5-cm) piece of fresh ginger root, peeled and thickly sliced
1 large garlic clove, thickly sliced
3 kaffir lime leaves, torn in half
2 lemon grass stalks, halved
handful of spinach or bok choy leaves
1/2 cup (50 g) bean sprouts
1–2 fresh red chilies, seeded and finely sliced
2 tablespoons fresh cilantro
1 tablespoon Thai fish sauce

To serve
lime wedges
chili sauce

1 Place the tofu on a plate covered with paper towel and allow to stand for 10 minutes to drain.

2 Heat the oil in a wok or skillet until hot, add the tofu, and cook for 2–3 minutes, stirring, or until the tofu is golden brown. Remove from the wok or skillet and drain on paper towels.

3 Meanwhile, soak the noodles in boiling water for 2 minutes, then drain.

4 Place the stock in a large saucepan. Add the ginger root, garlic, lime leaves, and lemon grass and bring to a boil. Reduce the heat, add the tofu, noodles, spinach or bok choy, bean sprouts, and chilies and heat through for a couple of minutes. Stir in the cilantro and the Thai fish sauce, then pour into warmed deep soup bowls to serve. Serve with lime wedges and chili sauce.

preparation time
10 minutes

cooking time
40 minutes

serves 4

nutritional values per serving
- 230 kcals
- 4 g fat
- 0.4 g saturated fat
- 12 g fiber
- Source of phytoestrogens

Cook's tip
Rinsing canned beans will help to remove some of the sugars that can cause gas. Vitamin C in an accompanying glass of fruit juice will help your body absorb the iron from the beans.

Tuscan bean soup

1 tablespoon olive oil
1 small red onion, finely chopped
1 garlic clove, finely chopped
1 carrot, diced
2 celery stalks, chopped
1½ cups (400 g) canned chopped tomatoes
1 tablespoon sun-dried tomato paste
2½ cups (600 ml) vegetable stock
3 cups (750 g) canned mixed beans, drained and rinsed
3 tablespoons chopped flat-leaf parsley
salt and freshly ground black pepper
ready-made fresh pesto, to serve

1 Heat the oil in a heavy saucepan and sauté the onion for about 5 minutes, or until softened. Stir in the garlic, carrot, and celery and continue to cook for a further 5 minutes.

2 Add the tomatoes, tomato paste, stock, and seasoning. Bring to a boil, then reduce the heat and simmer, stirring occasionally, for 20–30 minutes, or until the vegetables are soft.

3 Place half of the vegetable mixture into a blender or food processor and blend until smooth, then return to the saucepan. Add the beans and simmer for a further 10 minutes, or until the beans have been heated through. Just before serving, stir in the chopped parsley. Serve in warmed soup bowls, garnished with a spoonful of pesto.

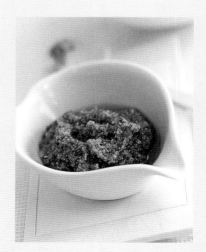

preparation time
15 minutes

cooking time
40 minutes

serves 2

nutritional values per serving
- 262 kcals
- 7 g fat
- 1 g saturated fat
- 5 g fiber
- Source of phytoestrogens

Cook's tip
Red lentils, often available in split form, do not need presoaking, only rinsing. Yellow lentils could be used in the same way instead.

curried lentil soup

1 tablespoon vegetable oil
1 small onion, finely chopped
1 garlic clove, crushed
1 small potato, finely diced
1 carrot, finely diced
2 celery stalks, finely chopped
1 tablespoon mild curry paste
1/2 cup (50 g) red lentils
3/4 cup (200 g) canned chopped tomatoes
2 1/2 cups (600 ml) chicken or vegetable stock
salt and freshly ground black pepper
chopped fresh cilantro, to garnish

1 Heat the oil in large saucepan, add the onion, and cook over a medium heat for 5 minutes, or until the onion begins to soften. Add the garlic, potato, carrot, celery, and curry paste and continue to cook, stirring occasionally, for a further 5 minutes.

2 Add the lentils, tomatoes, stock, and seasoning and bring the mixture to a boil. Reduce the heat, cover, and simmer for 30 minutes, or until the lentils are soft.

3 Garnish with a little chopped cilantro before serving.

preparation time
10 minutes

cooking time
20 minutes

serves 4

nutritional values per serving
- 250 kcals
- 12 g fat
- 4 g saturated fat
- 6 g fiber

pea, lettuce, and lemon soup with sesame croutons

2 tbsp (25 g) butter
1 large onion, finely chopped
3 cups (425 g) frozen peas
2 Bibb lettuces, roughly chopped
4$\frac{1}{4}$ cups (1 liter) vegetable or chicken stock
grated zest and juice of $\frac{1}{2}$ lemon
salt and freshly ground black pepper

Sesame croutons
2 thick slices of Miracle Bread (see page 132), cubed
1 tablespoon olive oil
1 tablespoon sesame seeds

1 To make the croutons, brush the bread cubes with the oil and place in a baking pan. Sprinkle with the sesame seeds and bake in a preheated oven at 400°F for 10–15 minutes, or until golden.

2 Meanwhile, heat the butter in a large saucepan, add the onion, and cook for 5 minutes or until the onion begins to soften. Add the peas, lettuce, stock, lemon zest, and juice and seasoning. Bring to a boil, then reduce the heat, cover, and simmer for 10–15 minutes.

3 Allow the soup to cool slightly, then transfer to a blender or food processor and puree until smooth. Return the soup to the saucepan, adjust the seasoning if necessary, and heat through. Spoon into warmed serving bowls and sprinkle with the sesame croutons.

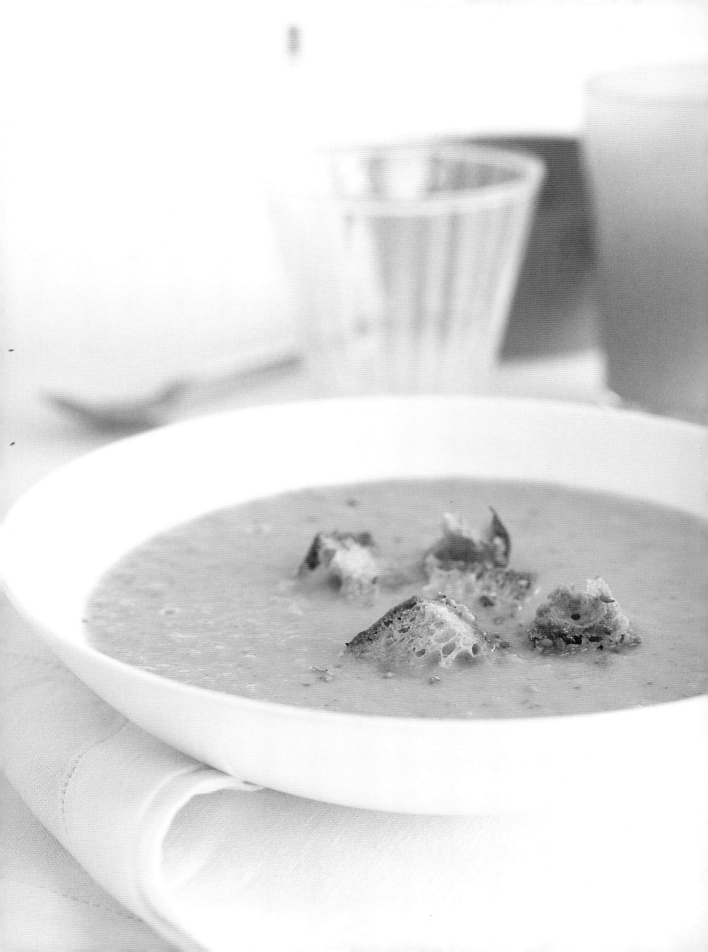

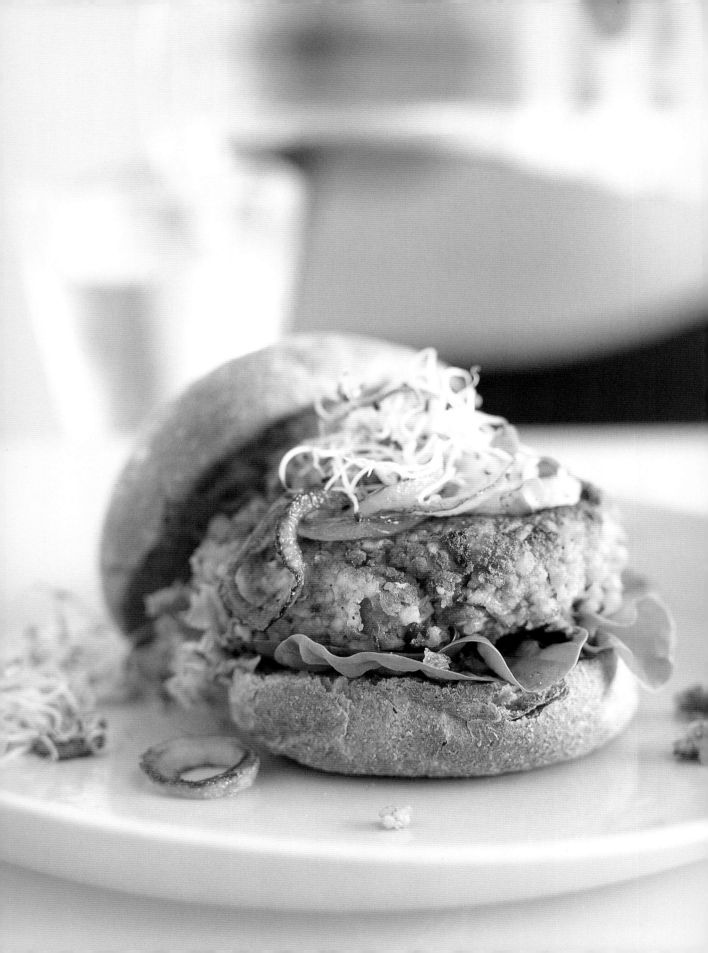

preparation time
15 minutes

cooking time
10–15 minutes

serves 4

nutritional values per serving
- 200 kcals
- 14 g fat
- 2 g saturated fat
- 2 g fiber
- Good source of phytoestrogens

curried tofu burgers

1 tablespoon vegetable oil, plus extra for sautéing
1 large carrot, coarsely grated
1 small red onion, finely chopped
1 garlic clove, crushed
1 teaspoon hot curry paste
1 teaspoon sun-dried tomato paste
8 oz (250 g) firm tofu, drained
1/2 cup (25 g) whole-wheat breadcrumbs
1/4 cup (about 25 g) unsalted peanuts, finely chopped
all-purpose flour, for dusting
vegetable oil, for frying
salt and freshly ground black pepper

Serve these spicy burgers in whole-wheat buns or pita bread with plenty of crisp lettuce and onion rings.

1 Heat the oil in a large, nonstick skillet. Add the carrot and onion and sauté for 3–4 minutes, or until the vegetables have softened, stirring constantly. Add the garlic and curry and tomato pastes. Increase the heat and sauté for 2 minutes, stirring all the time.

2 Place the tofu, vegetables, breadcrumbs, and nuts in a blender or food processor and process until just blended. Season well and beat until the mixture starts to stick together.

3 With floured hands, shape the mixture into 4 burgers. Heat a little oil in a large, nonstick skillet and fry the burgers for 3–4 minutes on each side, or until golden brown. Alternatively, to broil the burgers, brush them with a little oil and cook under a preheated hot broiler for about 3 minutes on each side, or until golden brown. Drain on paper towels and serve.

preparation time
15 minutes

cooking time
10 minutes

serves 2

nutritional values per serving
- 238 kcals
- 2 g fat
- 0.5 g saturated fat
- 14 g fiber
- Good source of phytoestrogens

spiced cannellini beans

2 teaspoons cumin seeds
1 red onion, finely chopped
about 8 tablespoons (1/2 cup) vegetable stock
1 green chili, seeded and finely chopped
2 garlic cloves, crushed
2 medium-sized (about 300 g) ripe tomatoes, peeled and chopped
2 tablespoons sun-dried tomato paste
1 1/2 cups (400 g) canned cannellini beans, drained and rinsed
2 1/2 cups (75 g) spinach leaves
salt and freshly ground black pepper
toasted Miracle Bread (see page 132), to serve

1 Toast the cumin seeds in a dry, heavy saucepan until fragrant, then add the onion and 2 tablespoons of the stock. Gently cook for 5 minutes, adding extra stock as necessary. Add the chili and garlic and dry-fry for a further 1 minute.

2 Stir in the tomatoes, tomato paste, beans, and 4 tablespoons of the stock. Bring to a boil, then reduce the heat and simmer for 5 minutes.

3 Season well and stir in the spinach, then remove from the heat. Stir until the spinach has just wilted. Serve with toast.

preparation time
15 minutes

cooking time
8–10 minutes

serves 2

nutritional values per serving
- 235 kcals
- 11 g fat
- 2 g saturated fat
- 2 g fiber
- Good source of phytoestrogens

tofu kebabs with barbecue sauce

2 tablespoons dark soy sauce
2 tablespoons tomato puree
2 tablespoons honey
1 tablespoon white wine vinegar
1 garlic clove, finely chopped
1 tablespoon sesame oil
8 oz (250 g) firm tofu, cut into
1-inch (2.5-cm) cubes
2 zucchini, sliced into
1-inch (2.5-cm) slices
6 green onions, cut into
2-inch (5-cm) lengths

1 To make the marinade, mix the soy sauce, tomato puree, honey, vinegar, garlic, and oil together in a large bowl. Brush the marinade over the tofu. Soak 4 bamboo skewers in cold water for 30 minutes.

2 Thread the tofu, zucchini, and green onions onto the skewers. Place the kebabs under a preheated hot broiler for 4–5 minutes, turn, and continue to cook for a further 4–5 minutes, or until cooked through and lightly charred.

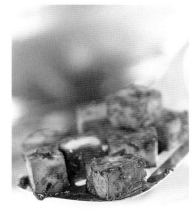

preparation time
15 minutes

cooking time
30 minutes

serves 2

nutritional values per serving
- 370 kcals
- 16 g fat
- 4 g saturated fat
- 9 g fiber
- Source of phytoestrogens

Cook's tip
For a speedier dish, replace the dry lentils with 2 cups (400 g) canned lentils. Rinse and drain the lentils, then start the recipe from Step 2.

lentils with fava beans, bacon, and poached egg

3/4 cup (about 75 g) brown lentils
1 thyme sprig
1 celery stalk
1 garlic clove
4 1/4 cups (1 liter) water
3 strips of smoked Canadian bacon, roughly chopped
1 tablespoon olive oil
4 green onions, finely sliced
2 1/2 cups (200 g) frozen fava beans, blanched and outer skins removed
1 tablespoon balsamic vinegar
2 eggs
salt and freshly ground black pepper

1 Place the lentils, thyme, celery, and garlic in a saucepan and pour over the measured water. Bring to a boil, then reduce the heat and simmer for 20 minutes or until tender. Drain the lentils and discard the thyme, celery, and garlic.

2 Fry the bacon in the oil for 2–3 minutes, then add the green onions and fava beans and fry for a further 2–3 minutes. Add the lentils and continue to cook for 1 minute. Season to taste and stir in the vinegar.

3 Meanwhile, poach the eggs in simmering water for just a couple of minutes. Remove with a slotted spoon and drain on paper towels. Divide the lentil mixture between 2 plates and top each mound with a poached egg. Serve immediately.

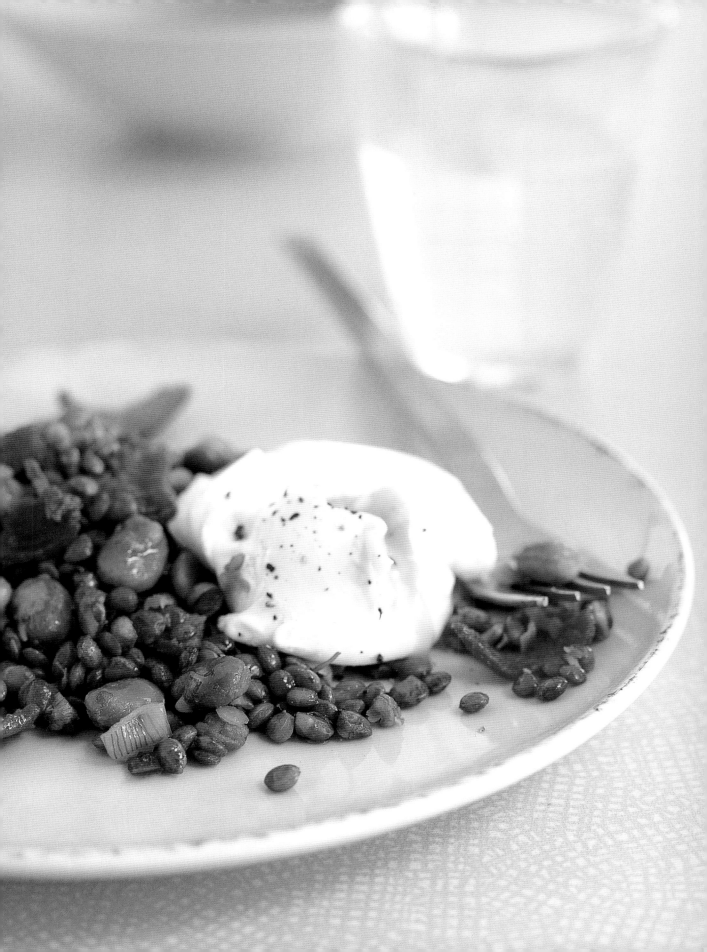

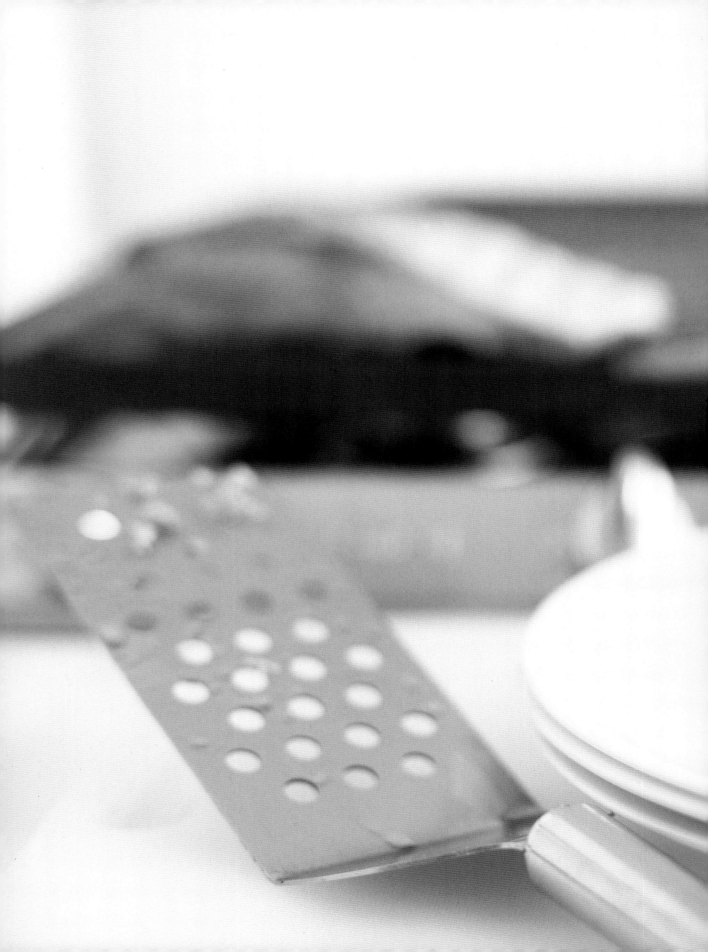

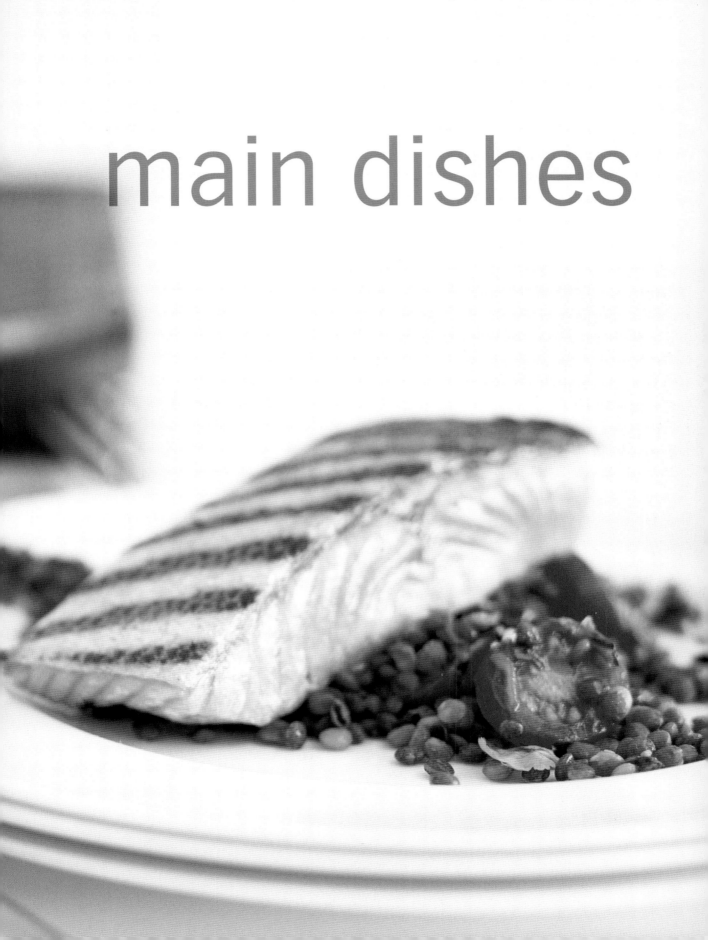

main dishes

preparation time
15 minutes

cooking time
30 minutes

serves 2

nutritional values per serving
- 500 kcals
- 23 g fat
- 6 g saturated fat
- 11 g fiber
- Source of phytoestrogens

Cook's tip
Use Miracle Bread (see page 132) or another bread rich in phytoestrogens to make the breadcrumbs.

spicy sausage cassoulet

1 tablespoon olive oil
1 red onion, finely chopped
1 garlic clove, crushed
1 red sweet pepper, cored, seeded, and roughly chopped
2 celery stalks, roughly chopped
3/4 cup (200 g) canned chopped tomatoes
1/2 cup (125 ml) chicken stock
2 teaspoons dark soy sauce
1 teaspoon Dijon-style mustard
1 1/4 cups (400 g) canned black-eyed peas, drained and rinsed
4 oz (125 g) low-fat smoked pork sausage, roughly chopped
1 cup (about 50 g) fresh breadcrumbs
1/4 cup (25 g) freshly grated Parmesan
2 tablespoons chopped parsley
salad made with crisp green lettuce, to serve

1 Heat 2 teaspoons of the oil in a large, nonstick skillet or wok, add the onion, garlic, red sweet pepper, and celery and cook over a low heat, stirring occasionally, for 3–4 minutes.

2 Add the tomatoes, stock, and soy sauce. Bring to a boil, then reduce the heat and simmer for about 15 minutes, or until the sauce begins to thicken. Add the mustard, beans, and sausage and continue to cook for a further 10 minutes.

2 Mix the breadcrumbs, Parmesan, and parsley together and sprinkle over the sausage mixture. Drizzle over the remaining oil and place under a preheated medium-hot broiler for 2–3 minutes, or until golden brown. Serve with a crisp green salad.

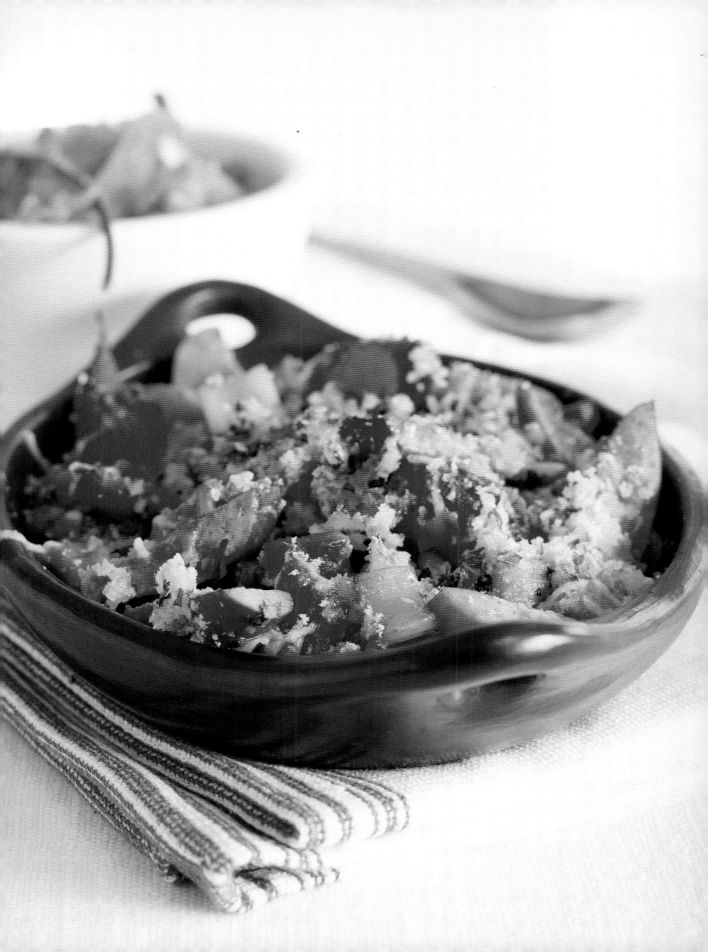

preparation time
15 minutes

cooking time
10–15 minutes

serves 2

nutritional values per serving
- 450 kcals
- 24 g fat
- 5 g saturated fat
- 2 g fiber
- Source of phytoestrogens

chicken and sesame goujons

1³/4 cups (75 g) fresh breadcrumbs
2 tablespoons sesame seeds
2 large skinless, boneless chicken breasts, cut into bite-sized pieces
1 egg, beaten
salt and freshly ground black pepper
olive oil spray
To serve
Spicy Red Sweet Pepper Dip
(see page 57)
crunchy mixed salad

1 Mix the breadcrumbs, sesame seeds, and seasoning together and spread over a large plate or baking pan. Dip the chicken pieces in the beaten egg, then roll in the breadcrumb mixture to coat thoroughly. Carefully lay the chicken on a lightly greased cookie sheet and chill for 30 minutes.

2 Spray the chicken pieces with the olive oil spray and cook in a preheated oven at 400°F for 10–15 minutes, or until the breadcrumbs are golden brown and the chicken is cooked through. Serve with Spicy Red Sweet Pepper Dip and a large crunchy salad.

preparation time
15 minutes

cooking time
30–35 minutes

serves 2

nutritional values per serving
- 490 kcals
- 14 g fat
- 4 g saturated fat
- 5 g fiber
- Source of phytoestrogens

chicken and lemon paella

4 teaspoons olive oil
10 oz (300 g) skinless, boneless
chicken thighs, diced
1 onion, sliced
2 garlic cloves, crushed
1 red sweet pepper, cored, seeded,
and roughly chopped
1/2 cup (about 75 g) easy-cook white
long-grain rice
2 tablespoons sherry
1 cup (250 ml) chicken stock
1 1/3 cups (200 g) frozen peas
grated rind and juice of 1 lemon
salt and freshly ground black pepper
thyme sprigs, to garnish
lemon wedges, to serve

1 Heat 2 teaspoons of the oil in a skillet over a medium heat and cook the chicken for 4–6 minutes, or until golden. Remove from the skillet and add the remaining oil. Add the onion and cook over a medium heat for 10 minutes until soft. Add the garlic and red sweet pepper and cook for a further 3 minutes.

2 Stir in the rice and pour in the sherry and stock. Return the chicken to the skillet. Turn the heat to low and cook for 10–15 minutes.

3 Add the peas and cook for a further 2–3 minutes, or until the liquid has evaporated. Stir in the lemon rind and juice, then season to taste. Serve garnished with thyme sprigs, accompanied by lemon wedges.

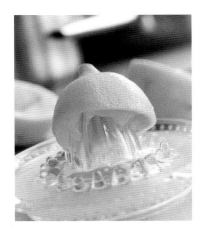

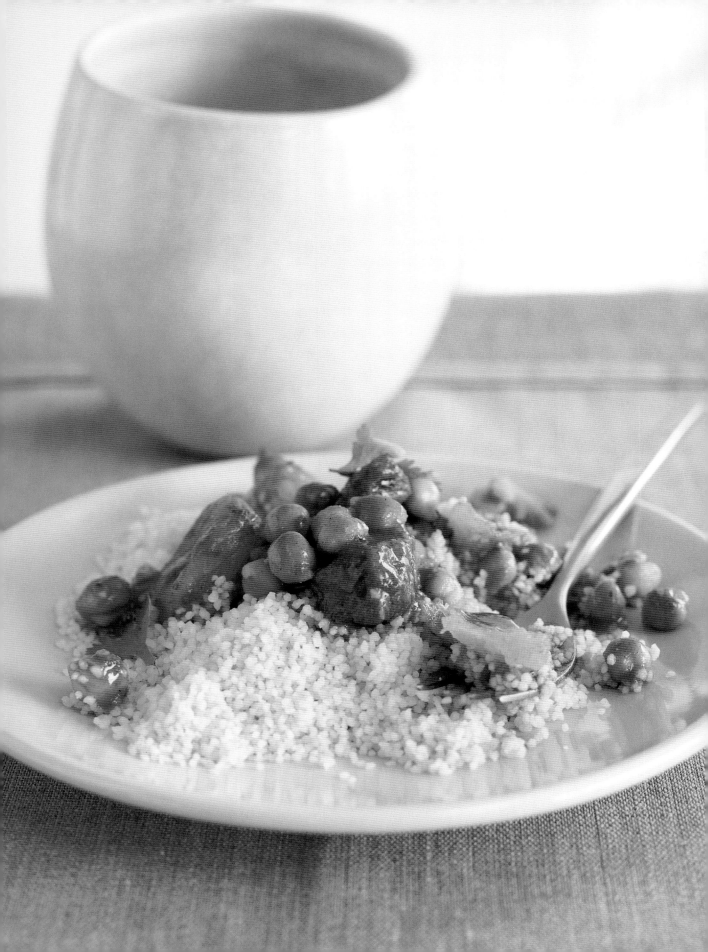

preparation time
15 minutes, plus marinating

cooking time
1¹⁄₂ hours

serves 2

nutritional values per serving
- 490 kcals
- 20 g fat
- 6 g saturated fat
- 8 g fiber
- Source of phytoestrogens

moroccan lamb

1 teaspoon dried ground ginger
1 teaspoon ground cumin
1 teaspoon paprika
1 cinnamon stick
¹⁄₄ cup (50 ml) orange juice
8 oz (250 g) lean lamb, cut into 2-inch
(5-cm) cubes
4 oz (125 g) pearl onions or shallots,
unpeeled
1 tablespoon olive oil
1 garlic clove, crushed
2 teaspoons flour
2 teaspoons tomato puree
¹⁄₂ cup (125 ml) lamb stock
3 tablespoons sherry
¹⁄₂ cup (about 50 g) dried apricots
1¹⁄₄ cup (300 g) canned chickpeas,
drained and rinsed
salt and freshly ground black pepper
couscous, to serve

1 Place the spices in a large bowl and pour over the orange juice. Add the lamb and mix well, cover, and leave in a cool place for at least 1 hour, or preferably overnight.

2 Place the onions or shallots in a saucepan of boiling water and cook for 2 minutes. Drain and refresh under cold water, then peel.

3 Heat the oil in a large flameproof casserole. Remove the lamb from the marinade and brown over a high heat until golden all over. Using a slotted spoon, remove the lamb and set aside. Reduce the heat slightly and, adding a little more oil if necessary, cook the onions or shallots and garlic for 3 minutes, or until just beginning to brown. Return the meat to the casserole and stir in the flour and tomato puree. Continue to cook for 1 minute.

4 Add the marinade to the casserole with the stock, sherry, and seasoning. Bring to a boil, then reduce the heat, cover, and place in a preheated oven at 350°F for 1 hour. Add the apricots and chickpeas and return to the oven for a further 15 minutes. Serve with couscous cooked according to the instructions on the package.

preparation time
15 minutes

cooking time
45 minutes

serves 2

nutritional values per serving
- 480 kcals
- 18 g fat
- 6g saturated fat
- 12 g fiber
- Good source of phytoestrogens

chilli con carne

1 tablespoon vegetable oil
1 red onion, finely chopped
1 garlic clove, finely chopped
8 oz (250 g) lean ground beef
1 small red sweet pepper, cored, seeded, and diced
1 1/2 cups (400 g) canned chopped tomatoes
1 tablespoon tomato puree
2 teaspoons chili powder
1 cup (about 200 ml) beef stock
1 1/2 cups (400 g) canned red kidney beans, drained and rinsed
salt and freshly ground black pepper
brown rice, to serve

1 Heat the oil in heavy, nonstick skillet. Add the onion and garlic and cook for 5 minutes, or until beginning to soften. Add the ground beef and cook for a further 5–6 minutes, or until browned all over.

2 Stir in the red sweet pepper, tomatoes, tomato puree, chili powder, and stock and bring to a boil. Reduce the heat and simmer gently for 30 minutes.

3 Add the beans and cook for a further 5 minutes. Season to taste and serve with brown rice, cooked according to the instructions on the package.

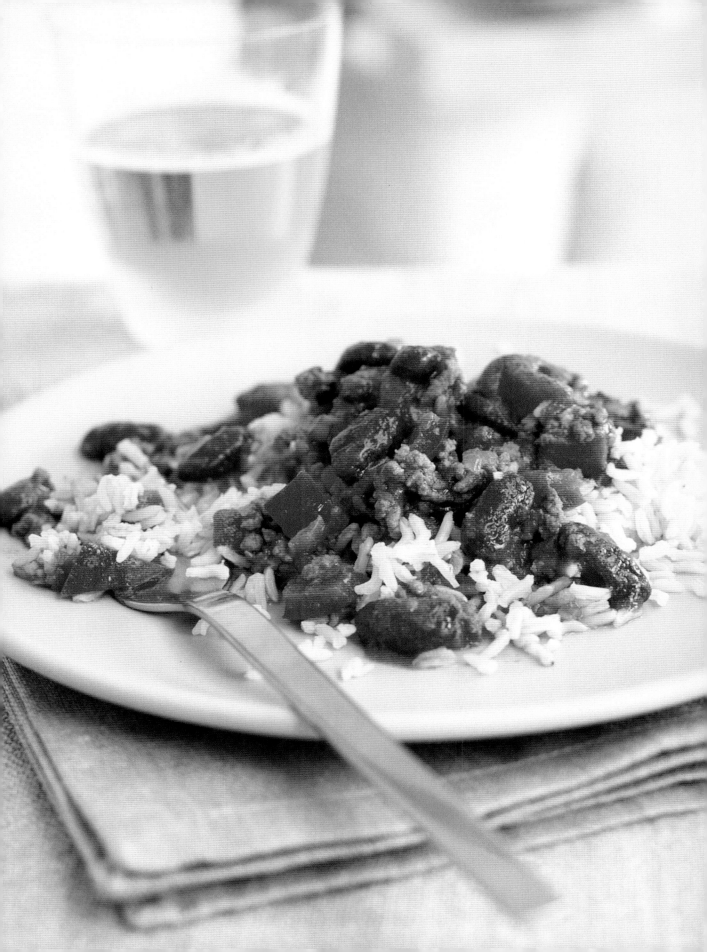

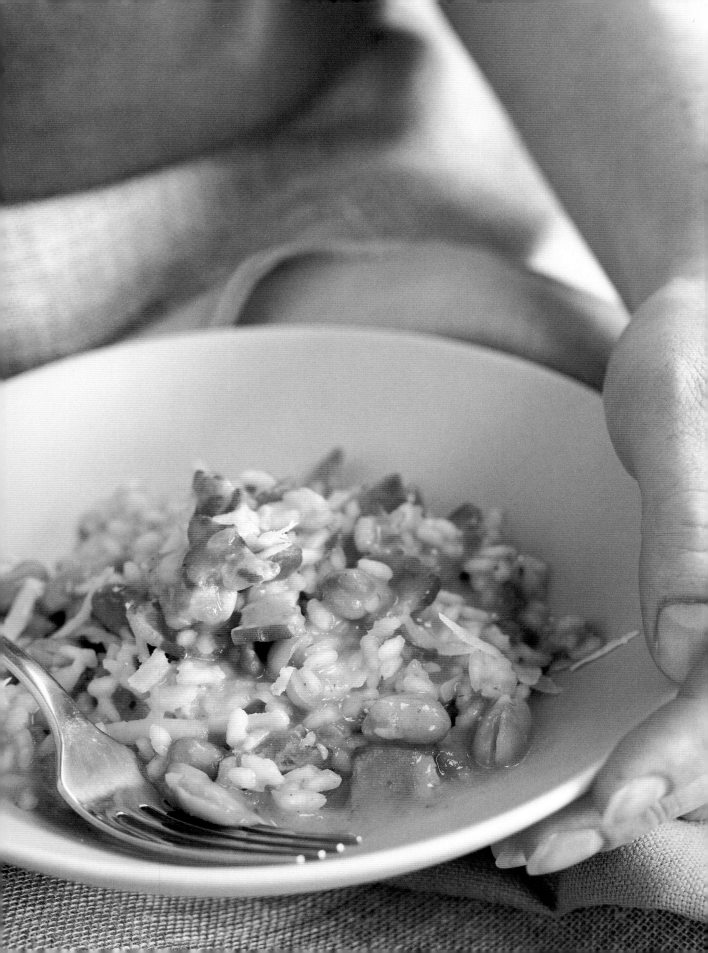

preparation time
15 minutes

cooking time
20 minutes

serves 2

nutritional values per serving
- 530 kcals
- 18 g fat
- 8 g saturated fat
- 10 g fiber
- Source of phytoestrogens

Cook's tip
Arborio rice is used to make risotto because it absorbs more liquid and releases more starch than other types of rice, producing a creamy, velvety result.

fava bean and bacon risotto

1²/3 cups (300 g) frozen fava beans
1 tbsp (15 g) butter
1 onion, finely chopped
4 strips of smoked Canadian bacon, rind removed, roughly chopped
²/3 cup (125 g) arborio rice
2¹/4 cups (500 ml) hot chicken stock
¹/4 cup (25 g) freshly grated Parmesan
salt and freshly ground black pepper
Parmesan shavings, to garnish

1 Cook the fava beans in a saucepan of lightly salted boiling water for 2–3 minutes. Drain and plunge into ice-cold water to cool. Peel away and discard the outer shells and set the beans aside.

2 Heat the butter in a heavy saucepan. Add the onion and bacon and cook over a low heat for 5 minutes. Add the rice and beans and continue to cook, stirring, for 1–2 minutes.

3 Add just enough hot stock to cover the rice and continue to cook, stirring frequently, until most of the stock has been absorbed. Continue adding the stock in this way until it is almost completely absorbed and the rice is tender.

4 Remove from the heat, stir in the grated Parmesan, and season to taste. Serve immediately, garnished with Parmesan shavings.

preparation time
10 minutes

cooking time
10–15 minutes

serves 2

nutritional values per serving
- 350 kcals
- 11 g fat
- 4 g saturated fat
- 9 g fiber
- Source of phytoestrogens

monkfish brochettes with cannellini beans and pesto

8 oz (250 g) monkfish, cut into 6 pieces
6 slices of Parma ham
6 cherry tomatoes
1 yellow sweet pepper, cored, seeded, and cut into 6 pieces
1 tablespoon olive oil
1¼ cups (300 g) canned cannellini beans, drained and rinsed
2 tablespoons ready-made fresh pesto

1 Wrap each piece of monkfish in a slice of Parma ham. Thread onto 2 skewers, alternating with tomatoes and yellow sweet pepper pieces. Brush the kebabs with the oil and cook under a preheated hot broiler for 3–4 minutes. Turn and broil for a further 3 minutes until cooked through.

2 Place the beans in a nonstick saucepan and cook, stirring, over a low heat for 4–5 minutes, or until hot. Stir in the pesto. Spoon the beans onto 2 plates, top with the brochettes, and serve immediately.

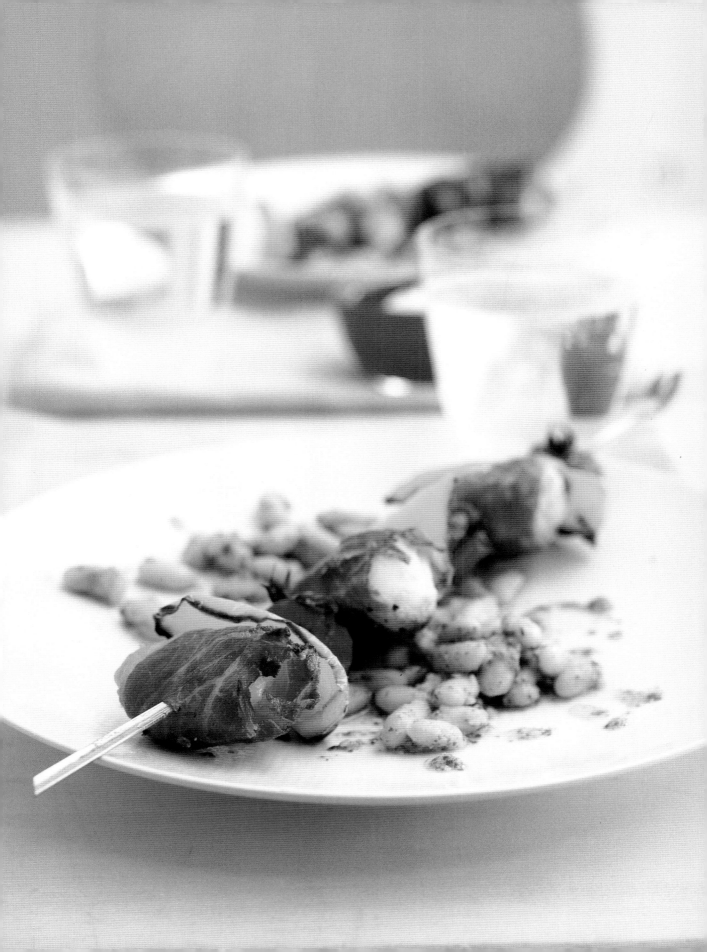

preparation time
15 minutes

cooking time
40–50 minutes

serves 2

nutritional values per serving
- 456 kcals
- 22 g fat
- 4 g saturated fat
- 6 g fiber
- Source of phytoestrogens

Cook's tip
If time is short, use a 2 cups (400 g) of canned lentils in place of the dried in Step 2. Add to the Worcestershire sauce, tomatoes, and cilantro.

seared salmon on a bed of lentils

1 tablespoon olive oil
1 small onion, finely chopped
1 garlic clove, finely chopped
1 fennel bulb, chopped
1/2 cup (100 g) brown lentils, washed
1 1/4 cups (300 ml) chicken or vegetable stock
1 tablespoon Worcestershire sauce
12 small cherry tomatoes, halved
3 tablespoons chopped fresh cilantro
2 5-oz (150-g) salmon fillets
salt and freshly ground black pepper

1 Heat the oil in a deep, nonstick skillet. Add the onion, garlic, and fennel and cook, stirring, for about 10 minutes, or until soft.

2 Add the lentils and stock and bring to a boil, then reduce the heat and simmer for 30–40 minutes, or until the lentils are tender. Stir in the Worcestershire sauce, tomatoes, and cilantro, and season to taste.

3 Meanwhile, cook the salmon fillets on a hot griddle or under a preheated hot broiler for about 4 minutes on each side, or until just cooked through. Spoon the lentils onto serving plates, top with the salmon fillets, and serve.

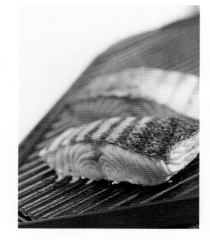

preparation time
15 minutes

cooking time
10–15 minutes

serves 2

nutritional values per serving
- 350 kcals
- 14 g fat
- 3 g saturated fat
- 7 g fiber
- Source of phytoestrogens

halibut with fava beans

1^1/$_3$ cups (200 g) fresh fava beans or
1^1/$_4$ cups (200 g) frozen fava beans
4 teaspoons olive oil
1 onion, chopped
4 strips of smoked Canadian bacon,
chopped
2 zucchini, cubed
1 garlic clove, finely chopped
8 canned artichoke hearts in brine,
drained and halved
handful of marjoram, chopped
handful of flat-leaf parsley, chopped
2 6-oz (175-g) halibut steaks
salt and freshly ground black pepper
lemon wedges, to garnish

1 Cook the fava beans in a saucepan of lightly salted boiling water for 4–5 minutes, or until just tender. Drain and plunge into ice-cold water to cool. Peel away and discard the outer shells and set the beans aside.

2 Heat 3 teaspoons of the oil in a nonstick skillet, add the onion and bacon, and cook for 5 minutes until softened. Add the zucchini and garlic and cook for a further 5 minutes, or until the zucchini are golden. Stir in the artichokes, herbs, and beans and continue to cook for 1–2 minutes, or until heated through. Season to taste.

3 Place the halibut steaks on a lightly oiled baking pan with low sides, brush with the remaining oil, and season to taste. Place under a preheated hot broiler and cook for 2–3 minutes on each side. Spoon the bean mixture onto 2 serving plates and arrange the fish on top. Serve immediately, garnished with lemon wedges.

preparation time
10 minutes

cooking time
4–6 minutes

serves 2

nutritional values per serving
- 570 kcals
- 28 g fat
- 6 g saturated fat
- 13 g fiber
- Source of phytoestrogens

Cook's tip
Don't be seduced by large, smooth-skinned varieties of avocado—the small, pebbly-textured Haas avocados have a creamier texture and better flavor.

griddled tuna with black-eyed pea and avocado salsa

1 large ripe avocado, halved, seeded, peeled, and diced
4 ripe plum tomatoes, quartered, seeded, and diced
1 small red onion, finely chopped
1¼ cups (300 g) canned black-eyed peas, drained and rinsed
2 tablespoons chopped fresh cilantro
finely grated zest and juice of 1 lime
2 5-oz (150-g) fresh tuna steaks
1 tablespoon olive oil
salt and freshly ground black pepper

1 To make the salsa, mix the avocado, tomatoes, onion, and peas together in a large bowl. Stir in the cilantro, lime zest, juice, and seasoning to taste. Set aside.

2 Brush the tuna steaks with the oil. Place on a hot griddle and sear for 2–3 minutes on each side, or until cooked to your liking. Transfer the tuna to warmed serving plates and serve with the salsa

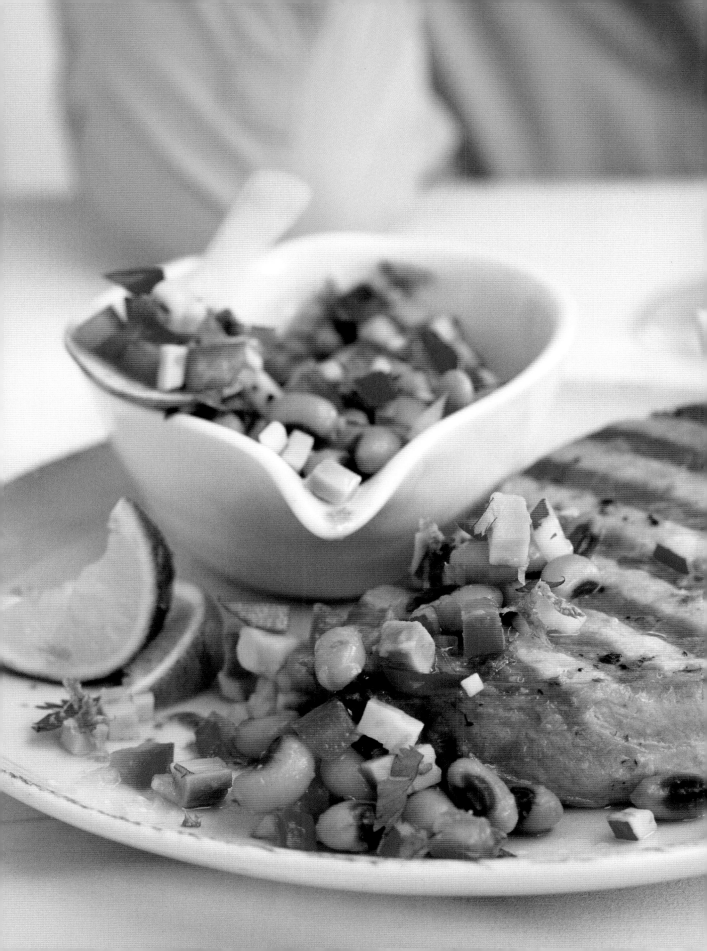

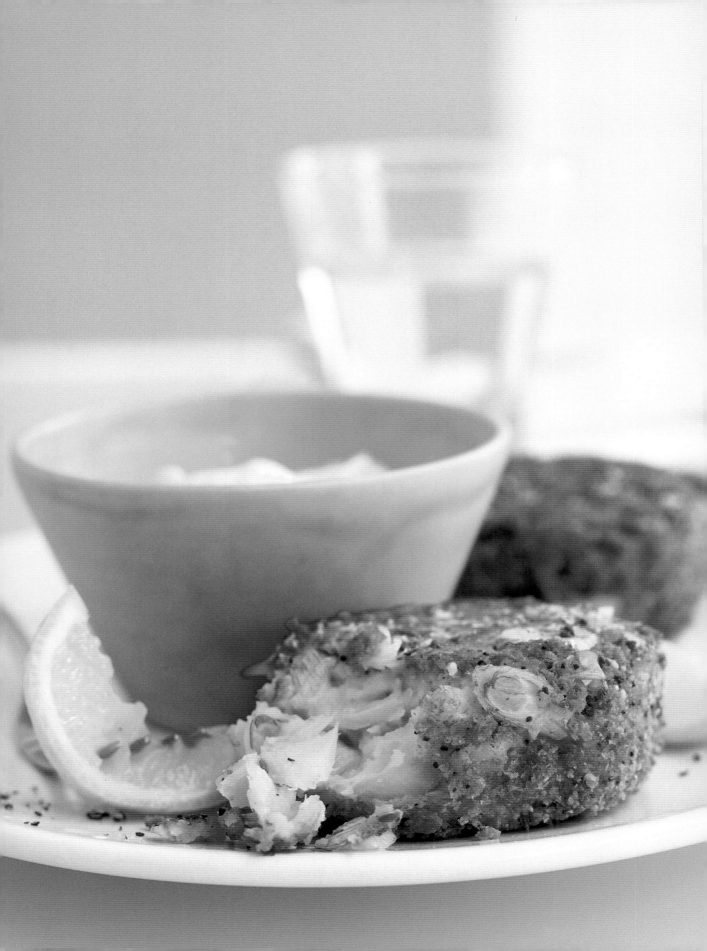

preparation time
20 minutes, plus chilling

cooking time
35 minutes

serves 2

nutritional values per serving
- 350 kcals
- 14 g fat
- 2 g saturated fat
- 2 g fiber
- Source of phytoestrogens

Cook's tip
Instead of frying the fishcakes, bake them in a preheated oven at 400°F for 20 minutes. Don't puree the potatoes in a food processor or they will be too sloppy.

smoked haddock fishcakes

5 oz (150 g) smoked haddock
8 oz (250 g) russet, purple, or round white potatoes, cut into large chunks
2 tablespoons plain soy yogurt or light cream
3 green onions, finely chopped
all-purpose flour, for dusting
1 egg, beaten
1 cup (about 50 g) fresh breadcrumbs, made from Miracle Bread (see page 132)
1 tablespoon vegetable oil
salt and freshly ground black pepper
To serve
lemon wedges
Tofu and Garlic Dip (see page 56)

1 Place the fish in a large, shallow skillet and pour over just enough water to cover. Bring to a boil, then reduce the heat, cover, and simmer for 8–10 minutes, or until tender. Flake the fish, discarding the skin and bones. Set aside.

2 Meanwhile, place the potatoes in a large saucepan of lightly salted water, bring to a boil, and cook for 15–20 minutes, or until tender. Drain well, add the soy yogurt or cream, and mash until smooth. Add the fish and green onions, mix well, and season to taste. Cover and chill for at least 30 minutes.

3 Turn the mixture out onto a lightly floured work surface and shape into 4 fishcakes. Carefully dip each fishcake into the beaten egg, then into the breadcrumbs, making sure they are evenly coated.

4 Heat half the oil in a large skillet and cook 2 fishcakes over a high heat for 4 minutes on each side, or until the breadcrumbs are golden brown. Drain on paper towels, then transfer to a warm oven while you cook the remainder. Serve with lemon wedges and Tofu and Garlic Dip.

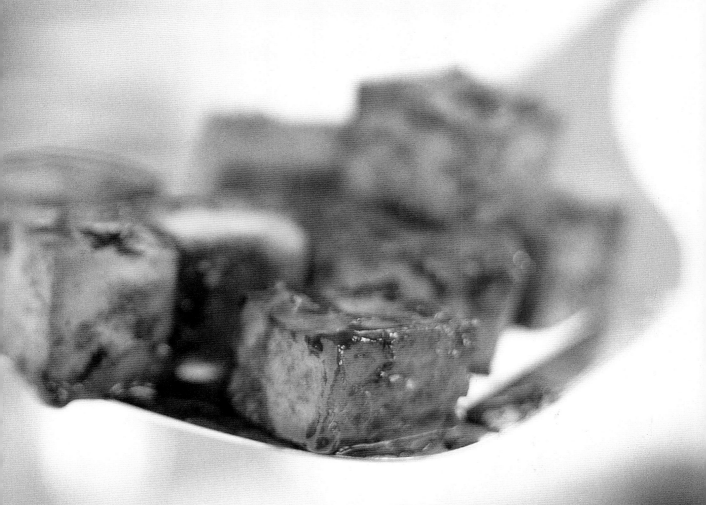

vegetarian
dishes

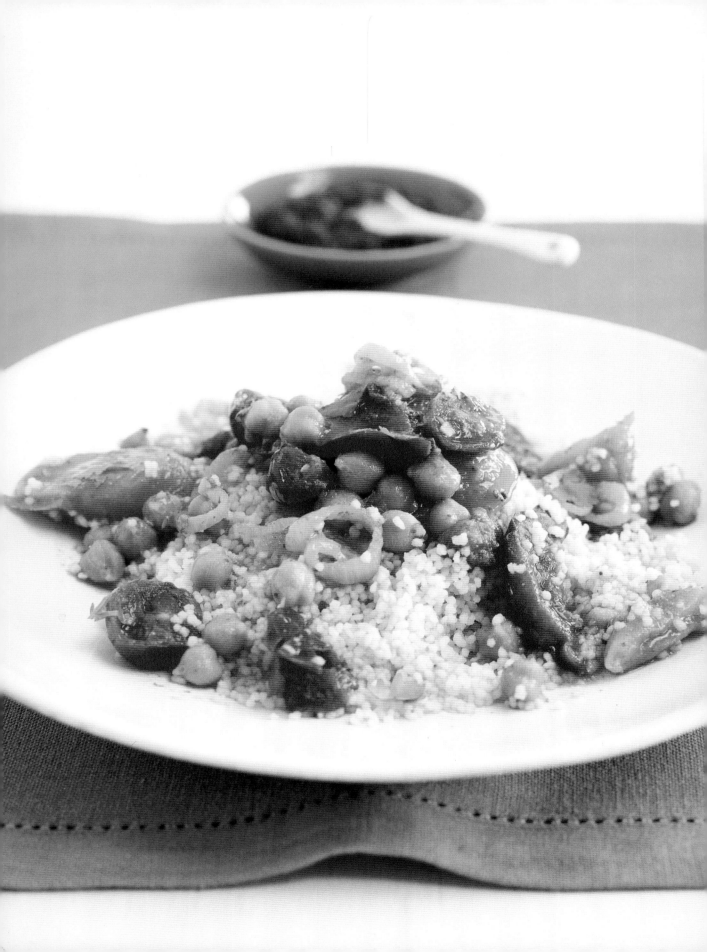

preparation time
15 minutes

cooking time
30 minutes

serves 2

nutritional values per serving
- 400 kcals
- 8 g fat
- 1 g saturated fat
- 13 g fiber
- Source of phytoestrogens

fragrant vegetable tagine

$1/2$ tablespoon olive oil
$1/2$ red onion, thinly sliced
1 garlic clove, crushed
dash of ground cumin
1 teaspoon harissa (chili paste)
$1/3$ cup (50 g) dried apricots, roughly chopped
1 large carrot, peeled and thickly sliced
$1/2$ red sweet pepper, cored, seeded, and roughly chopped
$3/4$ cup (200 ml) vegetable stock
$1 1/4$ cups (300 g) canned chickpeas, drained and rinsed
1 cup (about 125 g) cherry tomatoes, halved
1 tablespoon chopped fresh cilantro
1 tablespoon chopped mint leaves
salt and freshly ground black pepper
couscous, to serve

Serve this lightly spiced Moroccan stew with couscous for an authentic meal.

1 Heat the oil in a large saucepan, add the onion, and cook for 5 minutes, or until the onion begins to soften. Add the garlic, cumin, and harissa and cook for a further 1 minute.

2 Add the apricots, carrot, and red sweet pepper to the saucepan and stir. Pour over the stock and bring to a boil. Season to taste. Reduce the heat, cover, and simmer for 15 minutes.

3 Add the chickpeas and tomatoes and cook for a further 10 minutes, or until the vegetables are just tender. Stir in the cilantro and mint and serve with couscous.

preparation time
15 minutes, plus marinating

cooking time
10–15 minutes

serves 2

nutritional values per serving
- 450 kcals
- 31 g fat
- 6 g saturated fat
- 6 g fiber
- Good source of phytoestrogens

tofu kebabs with indonesian salad

1 garlic clove, minced

3 tablespoons dark soy sauce

1 teaspoon Barbados sugar

7 oz (200 g) firm tofu, drained and cut into 1-inch (2.5-cm) cubes

2 cups (about 125 g) white cabbage, shredded

1 carrot, peeled and julienned

1^3/$_4$ cups (175 g) bean sprouts

Satay sauce

1 tablespoon vegetable oil

1 garlic clove, crushed

1 teaspoon chili powder

^{1}/$_3$ cup (75 g) crunchy peanut butter

1 teaspoon Barbados sugar

^{2}/$_3$ cup (150 ml) water

1 Mix the garlic, soy sauce, and sugar together in a shallow dish and toss with the tofu. Cover and leave to marinate for at least 1 hour. Soak 4 bamboo skewers in cold water for 30 minutes.

2 To make the sauce, heat the oil in a saucepan and add the garlic and chili powder. Cook, stirring, for 1 minute. Add the peanut butter, sugar, and measured water. Bring to a simmer and cook for 4–5 minutes, or until the sauce thickens.

3 Meanwhile, blanch all the vegetables in boiling water for 2–3 minutes so that they do not lose their crunchiness. Drain well.

4 Thread the tofu onto the soaked skewers. Cook under a preheated hot broiler for 3–4 minutes on each side, or until browned. Serve the skewers on a mound of vegetables, with the satay sauce spooned over.

preparation time
10 minutes

cooking time
35 minutes

serves 2

nutritional values per serving
- 600 kcals
- 45 g fat
- 28 g saturated fat
- 2 g fiber
- Good source of phytoestrogens

Cook's tip
Thai green curry paste, available in most supermarkets, is a mild blend of spices including green chilies, lemon grass, coriander, garlic, kaffir lime leaves, and lime juice.

thai-spiced tofu with spinach

1 tablespoon vegetable oil
7 oz (200 g) firm tofu, drained and cut into 1-inch (2.5-cm) cubes
1 onion, peeled and finely chopped
2 teaspoons Thai green curry paste
1/2 cup (125 ml) coconut cream
1/2 cup (about 100 ml) vegetable stock
1 teaspoon Thai fish sauce (nam pla)
4 cups (125 g) fresh leaf spinach, roughly chopped
salt and freshly ground black pepper

Serve with Thai fragrant rice or boiled brown rice.

1 Heat the oil in a large, heavy skillet. Add the tofu and cook over a high heat for 2–3 minutes, or until golden. Add the onion and continue to cook for 2–3 minutes, or until softened. Stir in the curry paste and cook, stirring, for 1 minute.

2 Add the coconut cream, stock, and Thai fish sauce and bring to a boil. Reduce the heat, cover, and simmer over a low heat for 20 minutes.

3 Add the spinach in batches, stirring after each batch until it has wilted. Cook for a further 10 minutes. Season to taste before serving.

preparation time
15 minutes

cooking time
10 minutes

serves 2

nutritional values per serving
- 310 kcals
- 11 g fat
- 2 g saturated fat
- 1.5 g fiber
- Good source of phytoestrogens

Cook's tip
Tofu can be stored in the freezer for up to 3 months. If you can't find shiitake mushrooms use crimini mushrooms instead.

tofu with bok choy and shiitake mushrooms

4 teaspoons vegetable oil
7oz (200 g) firm tofu, drained and cut into 1-inch (2.5-cm) cubes
1 garlic clove, crushed
2 cups (about 150 g) shiitake mushrooms, roughly chopped
3 cups (200 g) bok choy, trimmed and roughly chopped
4 green onions, finely sliced
2 tablespoons plum sauce
2 tablespoons light soy sauce
2 tablespoons water
4 oz (125 g) rice noodles

1 Heat half the oil in a wok or skillet, add the tofu, and cook for 2–3 minutes, stirring, or until it is golden brown. Remove with a slotted spoon and set aside.

2 Heat the remaining oil in the skillet, add the garlic, mushrooms, bok choy, and green onions and cook for 2–3 minutes. Stir in the tofu, plum sauce, soy sauce, and measured water and cook for a further 2 minutes, or until the sauce is hot.

3 Cook the noodles according to the instructions on the package. Divide them between 2 bowls, spoon over the tofu mixture, and serve immediately.

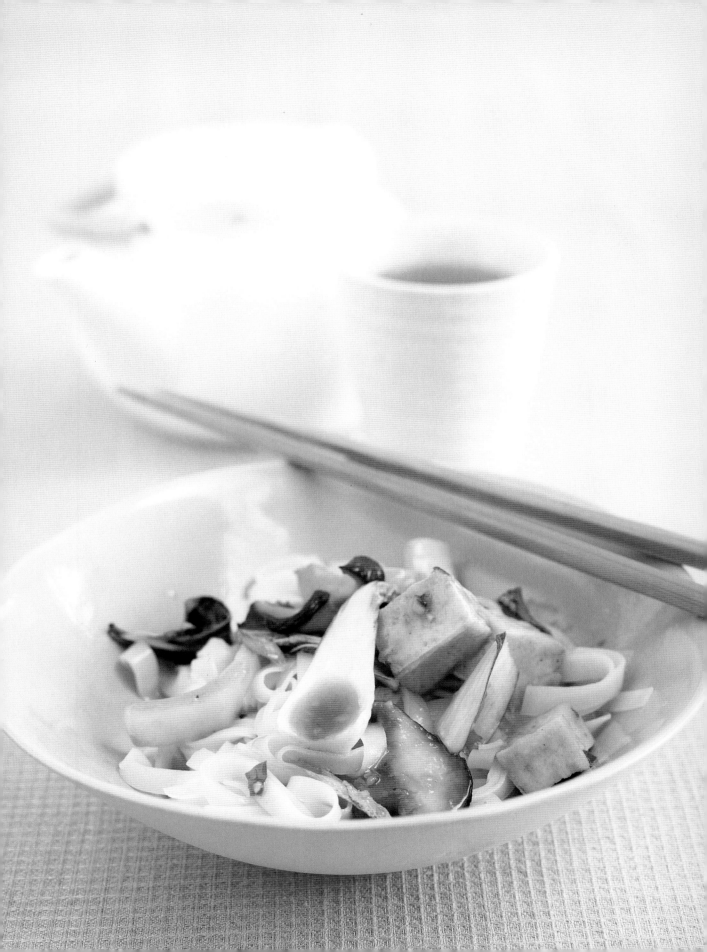

preparation time
20 minutes
cooking time
25 minutes

serves 2

nutritional values per serving
- 250 kcals
- 11 g fat
- 2 g saturated fat
- 7 g fiber
- Good source of phytoestrogens

roasted glazed tofu with stir-fried vegetables

7 oz (200 g) firm tofu
1 garlic clove, crushed
1 tablespoon hoisin sauce
1 tablespoon dark soy sauce
1 tablespoon sweet sherry vinegar
1 tablespoon sweet chili sauce
2 teaspoons honey
2 teaspoons sesame oil
1 tablespoon sunflower oil
1 red onion, roughly chopped
1 carrot, peeled and julienned
1 red sweet pepper, thinly sliced
1¾ cups (125 g) broccoli florets
1 cup (75 g) mushrooms, quartered
4 green onions, sliced
1 cup (75 g) snow peas
1½ cup (150 g) bean sprouts
2 tablespoons water
1 tablespoon toasted sesame seeds, to garnish

Serve this delicious tofu dish with boiled brown rice for a satisfying main meal.

1 Drain the tofu, cut into 1-inch (2.5-cm) cubes, and place in a shallow roasting pan. Mix the garlic, hoisin sauce, dark soy sauce, sherry vinegar, chili sauce, honey, and sesame oil together. Pour two-thirds of the mixture over the tofu and toss well to coat. Roast in a preheated oven at 425°F for 25 minutes, or until the tofu is deep golden brown and glazed, turning it over halfway through the cooking time.

2 Meanwhile, heat the sunflower oil in a wok or large skillet. Add the onion, carrot, red sweet pepper, broccoli, and mushrooms and stir-fry for 3 minutes. Add the green onions, snow peas, and bean sprouts and stir-fry for a further 2 minutes.

3 Add the measured water to the remaining glaze and pour it over the stir-fried vegetables. Cook for a further 2–3 minutes, or until the vegetables are just tender. Stir in the roasted tofu and serve topped with toasted sesame seeds.

preparation time
20 minutes,

cooking time
25 minutes

serves 6

nutritional values per serving
- 200 kcals
- 4 g fat
- 1 g saturated fat
- 8 g fiber
- Source of phytoestrogens

spicy bean burgers

1 tablespoon olive oil, plus extra for oiling
2 celery stalks, finely chopped
1 large red onion, finely chopped
1 large garlic clove, crushed
1 small red chili, seeded and finely chopped
1-inch (2.5-cm) piece of fresh ginger root, finely grated
3 1/2 cups (875 g) canned mixed beans
1 teaspoon ground cumin
2 tablespoons chopped fresh cilantro
all-purpose flour, for dusting
1 egg, beaten
2 cups (100 g) fresh breadcrumbs, made with Miracle Bread (see page 132)
salt and freshly ground black pepper

Tzatziki
1/2 cucumber
1 garlic clove, crushed
3/4 cup (about 200 ml) plain soy yogurt

1 To make the tzatziki, slice the cucumber in half lengthways and use a teaspoon to remove the seeds. Dice the flesh finely. Stir the cucumber and garlic into the soy yogurt and season lightly with salt and pepper.

2 Heat the oil in a nonstick skillet, add the celery, onion, garlic, chili, and ginger and cook over a medium heat for 5 minutes, or until softened.

3 Drain the beans, then rinse well and drain again. Place in a blender or food processor and pulse until almost smooth. Add the onion mixture, cumin, and cilantro and season to taste. Mix together well. Turn the mixture out onto a floured work surface and shape into 6 burgers. Cover and chill for 30 minutes.

4 Dip the burgers into the beaten egg, then carefully coat in breadcrumbs. Place on an oiled baking sheet and cook in a preheated oven at 400°F for 20 minutes. Serve immediately with the tzatziki.

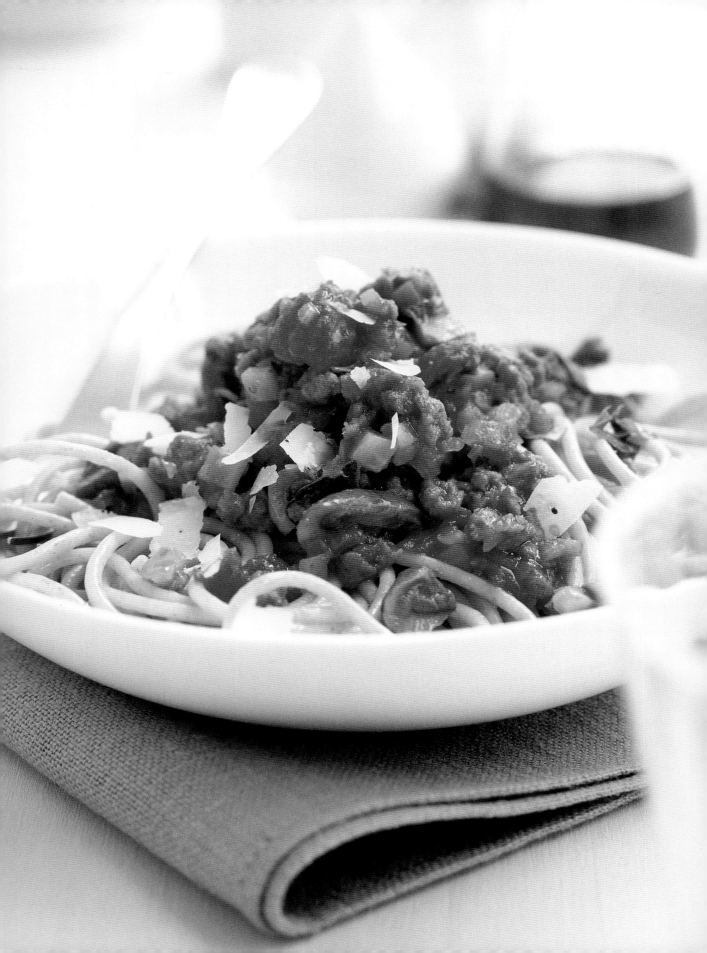

preparation time
15 minutes

cooking time
35–45 minutes

serves 2

nutritional values per serving
- 500 kcals
- 15 g fat
- 4 g saturated fat
- 8 g fiber
- Good source of phytoestrogens

spaghetti bolognese

1 tablespoon vegetable oil
1 onion, finely chopped
1 garlic clove, finely chopped
1 celery stalk, finely chopped
1 carrot, peeled and finely chopped
1 cup (75 g) crimini mushrooms, roughly chopped
1 tablespoon tomato puree
1 1/2 cups (400 g) canned chopped tomatoes
1 cup (about 250 ml) red wine or vegetable stock
dash of dried mixed herbs
1 teaspoon yeast extract
5 oz (150 g) textured vegetable protein (TVP)
2 tablespoons chopped parsley
7 oz (200 g) whole-wheat spaghetti
salt and freshly ground black pepper
freshly grated Parmesan, to serve

1 Heat the oil in a large, heavy saucepan. Add the onion, garlic, celery, carrot, and mushrooms and sauté for about 5 minutes, or until softened. Add the tomato puree and sauté for a further 1 minute.

2 Add the tomatoes, wine or stock, mixed herbs, yeast extract, and TVP. Bring to a boil, then reduce the heat, cover, and simmer for 30–40 minutes, or until the TVP is tender. Stir in the parsley and season to taste.

3 Cook the spaghetti in a saucepan of lightly salted boiling water for 12 minutes, or according to the package instructions. Drain well, then spoon onto serving plates. Top with the Bolognese mixture, sprinkle over a little Parmesan, and serve.

preparation time
15 minutes

cooking time
10–12 minutes

serves 2

nutritional values per serving
- 523 kcals
- 31 g fat
- 5 g saturated fat
- 7 g fiber
- Source of phytoestrogens

penne with fava beans and feta cheese

7 oz (200 g) penne or other pasta shapes
$1^{1}/_{3}$ cups (200 g) fresh fava beans or
$1^{1}/_{4}$ cups (200 g) frozen fava beans
2 oz (50 g) sun-dried cherry tomatoes
in oil, drained and roughly chopped
handful of mixed herbs, such as
parsley, tarragon, chervil, and chives,
roughly chopped
$1/_{2}$ cup (50 g) feta cheese, crumbled or
roughly chopped
salt and freshly ground pepper
Dressing
2 tablespoons extra virgin olive oil
1 tablespoon sherry vinegar
$1/_{2}$ teaspoon prepared whole-grain
mustard

1 Cook the penne for 10–12 minutes in a saucepan of lightly salted boiling water, or according to the instructions on the package. Refresh in cold water and drain well. Meanwhile, cook the fava beans in a separate saucepan of lightly salted boiling water for 4–5 minutes, or until just tender. Drain and plunge into ice-cold water to cool. Peel away and discard the outer shells.

2 Whisk the dressing ingredients together in a small bowl and season to taste with salt and pepper.

3 Place the beans in a serving dish and stir in the pasta, tomatoes, and herbs. Toss with the dressing. Season with freshly ground black pepper and sprinkle over the feta.

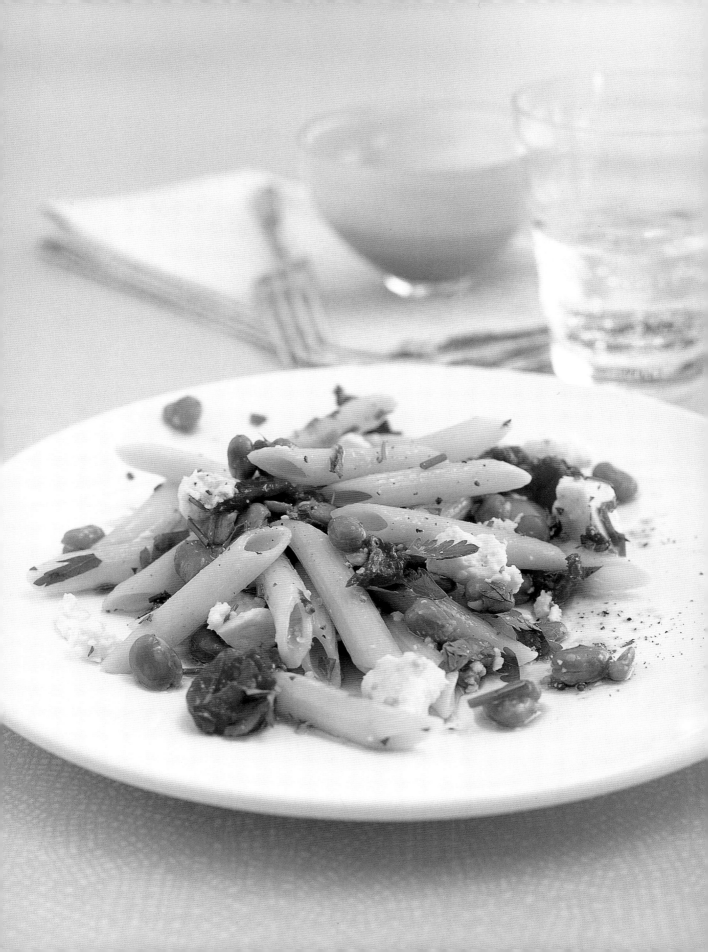

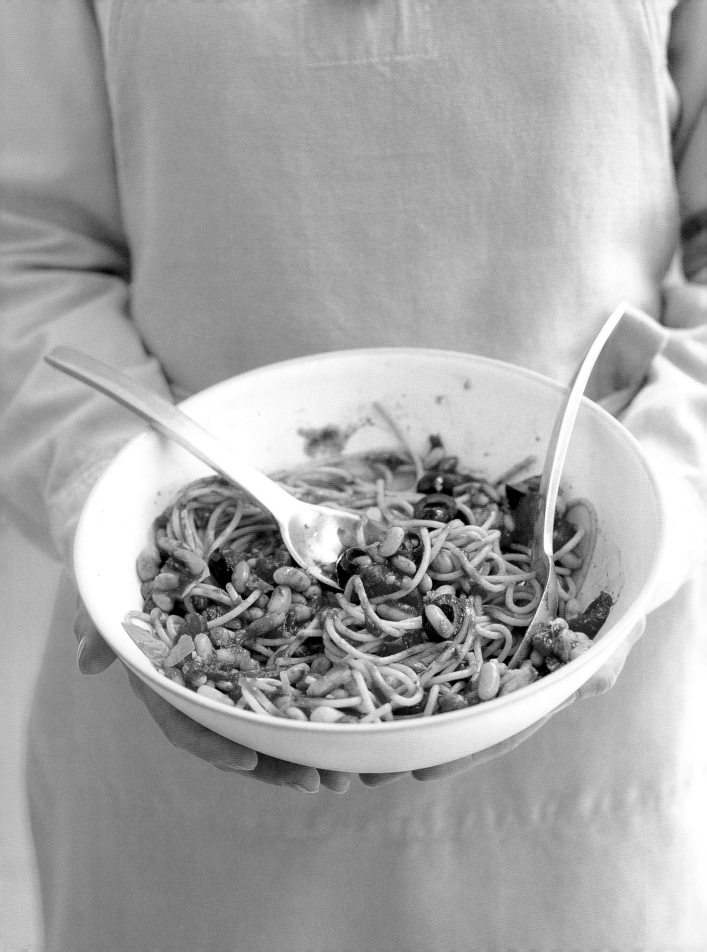

preparation time
10 minutes

cooking time
25 minutes

serves 2

nutritional values per serving
- 441 kcals
- 13 g fat
- 1.5 g saturated fat
- 14 g fiber

Cook's tip
The easiest way to make Parmesan shavings is to use a vegetable peeler.

spaghetti puttanesca

1 tablespoon olive oil
1 garlic clove, crushed
pinch of chili flakes
1 1/2 cups (400 g) canned chopped tomatoes
1/3 cup (50 g) pitted black olives, roughly chopped
1 tablespoon tomato puree
1 tablespoon capers
1 1/4 cups (300 g) canned flageolet beans, drained and rinsed
4 oz (125 g) whole-wheat spaghetti
handful of basil leaves
salt and freshly ground black pepper
Parmesan shavings, to serve

1 Heat the oil in a nonstick skillet. Add the garlic and chili flakes and cook for 3–4 minutes. Add the tomatoes, olives, tomato puree, capers, and beans. Reduce the heat and simmer for 20 minutes, or until the sauce is thick. Season to taste.

2 Meanwhile, cook the spaghetti for 10–12 minutes in a saucepan of lightly salted boiling water, or according to the instructions on the package.

3 Drain the pasta and return to the saucepan. Sir in the sauce and the basil and toss well. Sprinkle over the Parmesan shavings and serve.

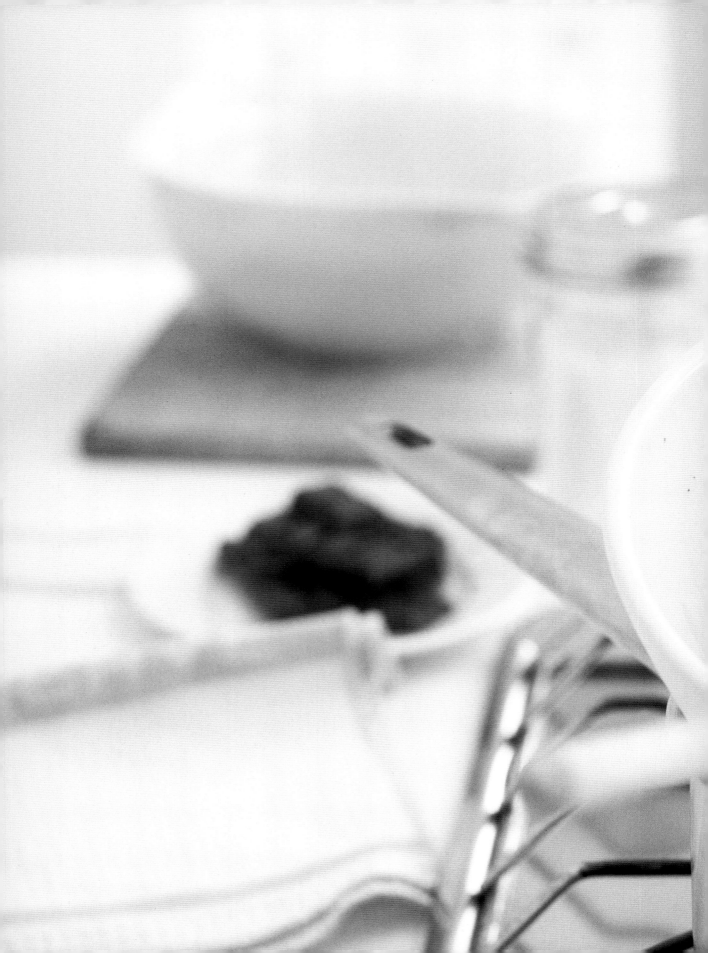

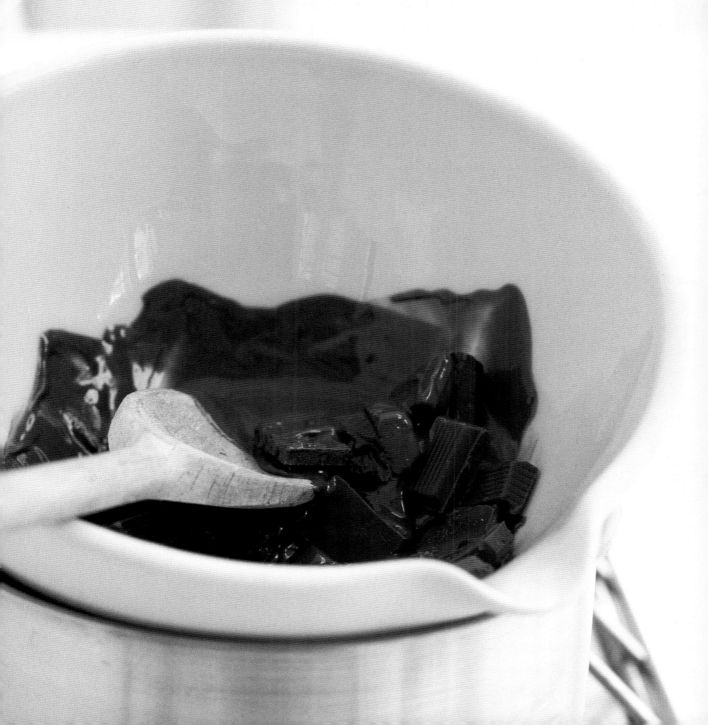

desserts

preparation time
10 minutes, plus freezing

cooking time
15 minutes

serves 4

nutritional values per serving
- 380 kcals
- 23 g fat
- 7 g saturated fat
- 0 g fiber

chocolate ice cream

2$1/4$ cups (500 ml) vanilla-flavored soy milk
1 cup (250 ml) soy cream
$1/4$ cup (50 g) sugar
3 large egg yolks
4 oz (125 g) semisweet chocolate, broken into pieces

1 Heat the soy milk and soy cream in a heavy saucepan until just below boiling point. Whisk the sugar and eggs yolks together in a large bowl until pale and thickened. Pour the hot liquid over the egg and sugar mixture, whisking all the time, then return the mixture to the saucepan. Place over a low heat and, stirring constantly, allow the mixture to thicken until it will just coat the back of a wooden spoon.

2 Remove from the heat and pour into a large, clean bowl. Add the chocolate and stir well. Allow the mixture to cool, then pour it into an ice-cream machine and churn until the mixture becomes thick and frozen. If you don't have an ice-cream machine, transfer the mixture to a shallow, freezerproof container. Freeze for at least 1 hour, or until the mixture is just beginning to set around the edges. Remove the container from the freezer and beat the mixture until smooth, then return to the freezer. Freeze for a further 30 minutes, then beat again. Repeat the freezing and beating process several more times until completely frozen.

3 Allow the ice cream to soften in the refrigerator for 2 hours before serving. Any leftovers will keep for up to 4 weeks in the freezer.

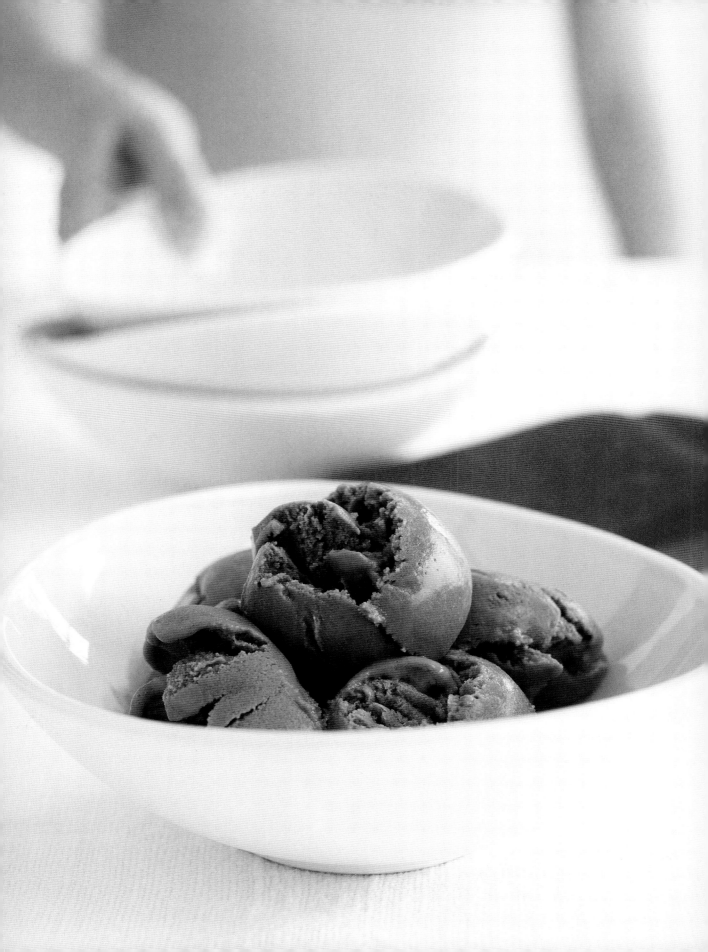

preparation time
10 minutes, plus chilling

cooking time
5 minutes

serves 2–3

nutritional values per serving
- 465–310 kcals
- 24–16 g fat
- 12–8 g saturated fat
- 0 g fiber
- Good source of phytoestrogens

mocha pudding

3 oz (75 g) milk chocolate,
broken into pieces
9 oz (250 g) silken tofu
2 teaspoons instant coffee mixed
with 1 teaspoon boiling water
$1/2$ cup (75 g) sour cream
$1/4$ cup (50 g) sugar
1 teaspoon vanilla extract
$1/2$ teaspoon ground cinnamon

1 Place the chocolate in a double boiler over gently simmering water. Allow the chocolate to melt, stirring from time to time.

2 Drain the tofu, place in a blender or food processor, and process until smooth. Add the chocolate, coffee mixture, sour cream, sugar, vanilla extract, and cinnamon and blend until creamy. Transfer to individual serving dishes. Chill thoroughly before serving.

preparation time
10 minutes, plus freezing

serves 2

nutritional values per serving
- 180 kcals
- 6 g fat
- 1g saturated fat
- 1 g fiber
- Source of phytoestrogens

banana and cardamom yogurt

1 large ripe banana, roughly chopped
1¼ cups (300 ml) plain soy yogurt
1 cardamom pod, seeds removed
and crushed
2 teaspoons honey (optional)
raspberries, to serve

1 Place the banana, soy yogurt, cardamom seeds, and honey, if using, in a blender or food processor and puree until smooth. Divide the mixture between 2 freezerproof bowls and transfer to the freezer for 1 hour.

2 Serve the yogurt with raspberries.

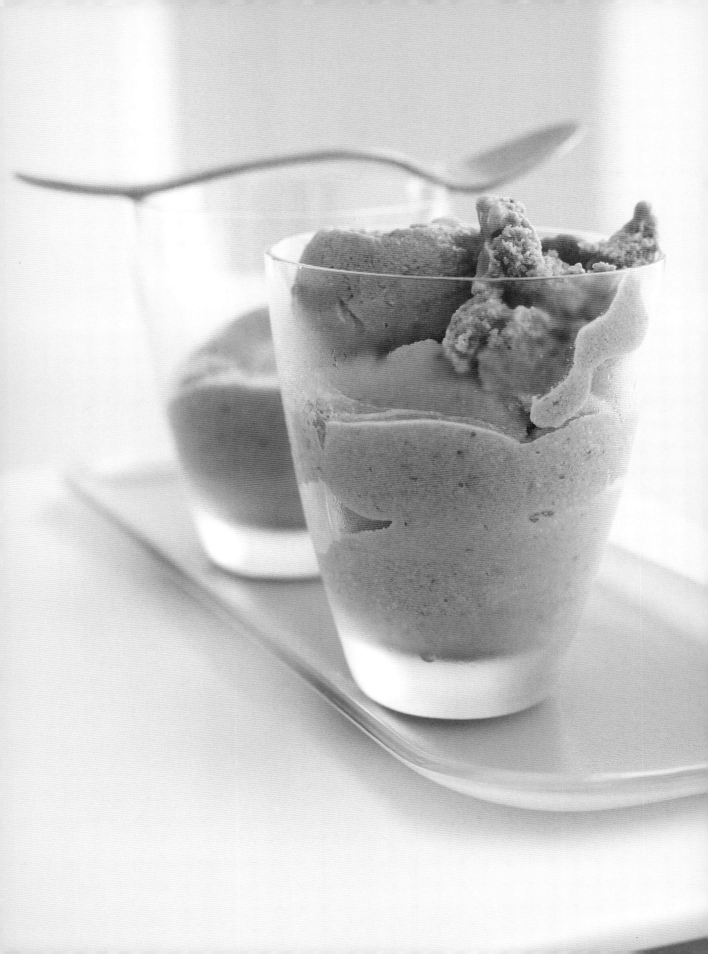

preparation time
15 minutes, plus freezing

cooking time
2 minutes

serves 2–3

nutritional values per serving
- 206–140 kcals
- 6–4 g fat
- 1–0.5 g saturated fat
- 1.5–1 g fiber
- Source of phytoestrogens

frozen strawberry yogurt

1²/₃ cups (250 g) strawberries, roughly chopped, plus extra to serve
2 tablespoons Concord grape juice
1 tablespoon crème de cassis
2 tablespoons powdered sugar
1¹/₄ cups (300 ml) soy yogurt

1 Place the chopped strawberries in a saucepan. Add the grape juice and warm gently, stirring occasionally, until the strawberries become soft and pulpy. Press the strawberries through a sieve and collect their juice in a large bowl. Discard the seeds. Beat in the crème de cassis, powdered sugar, and soy yogurt.

2 Pour the mixture into an ice-cream machine and churn until the mixture becomes thick and frozen. If you don't have an ice-cream machine, transfer the mixture to a shallow, freezerproof container. Freeze for at least 1 hour, or until the mixture is just beginning to set around the edges. Remove the container from the freezer and beat the mixture until smooth, then return to the freezer. Freeze for a further 30 minutes, then beat again. Repeat the freezing and beating process several more times until completely frozen.

3 Store in the freezer for up to 2 weeks. Transfer from the freezer to the refrigerator 20 minutes before serving.

preparation time
time 5 minutes, plus soaking

cooking time
3 minutes

serves 2–3

nutritional values per serving
- 164–110 kcals
- 0 g fat
- 0 g saturated fat
- 5–3 g fiber

dried fruit compote

1 cup (150 g) mixed dried fruit, such as apricots, apples, and prunes
1¼ cups (300 ml) orange or mango juice
1 cup (200 ml) boiling water
2 teaspoons arrowroot
1 cup (250 g) plain soy yogurt, to serve

1 Place the dried fruit in a large, heatproof bowl. Pour over the juice and the boiling water. Allow to cool, cover, and leave overnight in the refrigerator.

2 Mix the arrowroot with enough cold water to make a smooth paste. Drain the liquid from the fruit and place in a small saucepan, stir in the arrowroot paste, and bring to a boil. Cook for 1 minute, or until thickened, then pour over the compote. Set aside and leave to cool. Serve with soy yogurt.

preparation time
10 minutes

cooking time
20 minutes

serves 2

nutritional values per serving
- 245 kcals
- 8 g fat
- 4 g saturated fat
- 2 g fiber
- Source of phytoestrogens

apple custard

1 large cooking apple, such as a
Cortland, peeled, cored, and sliced
2 tablespoons sugar
2 tablespoons water
1 heaped tablespoon custard powder
1 cup (about 250 ml) vanilla-flavored
soy milk
1/2 cup (125 ml) strained plain yogurt
toasted sliced almonds, to decorate

1 Place the apple slices, half the sugar, and the measured water in a small saucepan. Cover and cook over a low heat for 10 minutes, or until soft. Beat with a wooden spoon to make a thick puree.

2 Place the custard powder and remaining sugar in a heatproof bowl and mix to a smooth paste with a little of the soy milk. Bring the remainder of the milk almost to a boil in a saucepan, pour onto the custard powder, and mix well. Return the mixture to the saucepan and bring to a boil, then reduce the heat and simmer for 1 minute, stirring constantly, until thick.

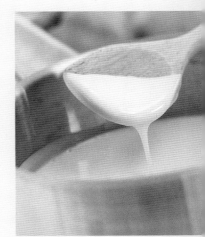

3 Allow the custard to cool, then stir in the pureed apple and yogurt and mix well. Spoon into serving dishes and chill. Decorate with toasted almond slices before serving.

preparation time
5 minutes

cooking time
5 minutes

serves 2

nutritional values per serving
- 50 kcals
- 0 g fat
- 0 g saturated fat
- 2 g fiber

summer fruit compote

2 cups (250 g) mixed summer fruit, such as raspberries, blueberries, and strawberries, thawed if frozen
finely grated zest and juice of 1 large orange
1 tablespoon redcurrant jelly
1 cup (250 g) plain soy yogurt, to serve

1 Place the fruit, orange zest and juice, and redcurrant jelly in a large saucepan. Cover and cook gently for 5 minutes, or until the juices flow and the fruit has softened. Remove from the heat and set aside. Chill and serve with soy yogurt.

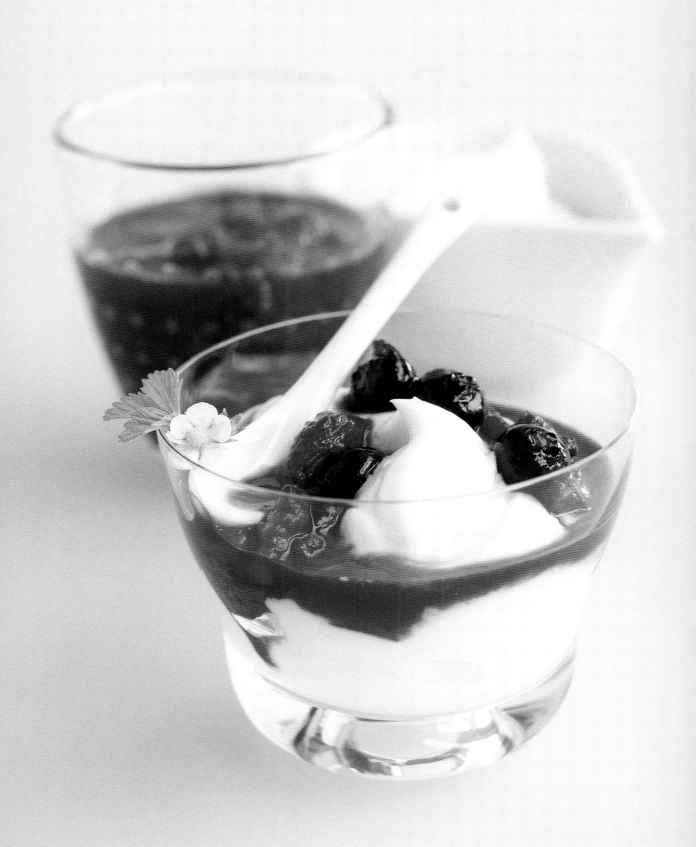

preparation time
10 minutes, plus chilling

cooking time
5 minutes

serves 2

nutritional values per serving
- 41 kcals
- 0 g fat
- 0 g saturated fat
- 2 g fiber

Cook's tip
If the remaining mixture sets before the final step, place it in a double boiler over gently simmering water until it becomes liquid again.

individual blueberry and elderflower molds

3 tablespoons elderflower cordial
2½ cups (600 ml) water
2 gelatin leaves
1 cup (125 g) blueberries

1 Mix the elderflower cordial with the measured water. Place 4 tablespoons of the mixture in a heatproof bowl, add the gelatin, and leave to soak for 5 minutes. Place the bowl over a pan of simmering water (or use a double boiler) and stir until it has dissolved. Stir the mixture into the remaining elderflower cordial mixture.

2 Divide the fruit between 2 large glasses, pour in enough of the liquid to just cover the fruit, then chill for about 30 minutes, or until just set.

3 Pour on the remaining liquid and chill for 3 hours, or until completely set.

preparation time
10 minutes

cooking time
25 minutes

serves 2

nutritional values per serving
- 328 kcals
- 14 g fat
- 5 g saturated fat
- 3 g fiber
- Good source of phytoestrogens

apricot risotto

3/4 cup (200 g) canned apricots in natural juice, drained
$1^2/3$ cups (400 ml) vanilla-flavored soy milk
1 tablespoon sugar
1 tbsp (15 g) butter
1/4 cup (50 g) arborio rice
1/4 cup (50 g) dried apricots, roughly chopped
2 tablespoons toasted sliced almonds, to decorate

1 Place the canned apricots in a blender or food processor and puree until smooth. Place the soy milk and sugar in a saucepan and heat gently, stirring occasionally, until the milk reaches simmering point. Reduce the heat to very low and allow the milk to simmer.

2 Melt the butter in large saucepan, add the rice, and cook, stirring, for 1–2 minutes. Add the dried apricots and cook for a further 1–2 minutes.

3 Add a ladleful of the warm milk and cook, stirring continuously, until the liquid is absorbed. Continue adding the milk in the same way until all the milk is used and the rice is tender—it will take about 20 minutes. Stir in the pureed apricots, then spoon into bowls and decorate with toasted flaked almonds.

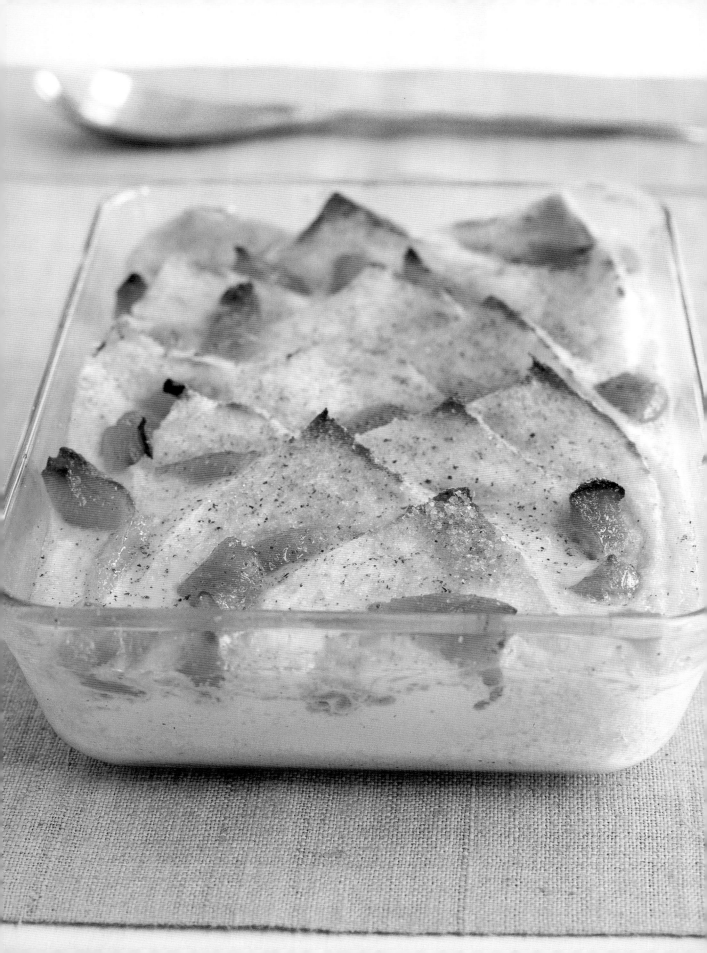

preparation time
10 minutes, plus standing

cooking time
30 minutes

serves 4

nutritional values per serving
- 420 kcals
- 16 g fat
- 8 g saturated fat
- 3 g fiber
- Source of phytoestrogens

bread and butter pudding

5 thick slices of white bread
3 tbsp (40 g) butter
$2/3$ cup (125 g) dark or golden raisins
3 eggs, beaten
$3^1/4$ cups (750 ml) vanilla-flavored soy milk
$1/4$ cup (50 g) sugar
1 tablespoon Demerara sugar, plus extra for sprinkling
dash of grated nutmeg

1 Remove the crusts from the bread, thinly spread with butter, then cut into triangles. Place half the bread in the bottom of a buttered $2^1/2$-pint (1.5-liter) shallow, ovenproof dish. (You could also use a 9x1$^1/2$-inch round cake pan.) Sprinkle over the dried fruit and arrange the remaining bread on top, buttered-side uppermost.

2 Beat the eggs, soy milk, and sugars together in a bowl. Strain the mixture , then pour over the bread. Allow to stand for 15 minutes.

3 Place the dish in a large roasting pan and pour enough hot water into the pan to come halfway up the sides of the dish. Sprinkle with the nutmeg and a little extra Demerara sugar and cook in a preheated oven at 350°F for 30 minutes, or until set and the top is crisp and golden. Serve immediately.

Variation
For a pudding with a nuttier texture, which is richer in phytoestrogens, use Miracle Bread (see page 132) instead of white bread.

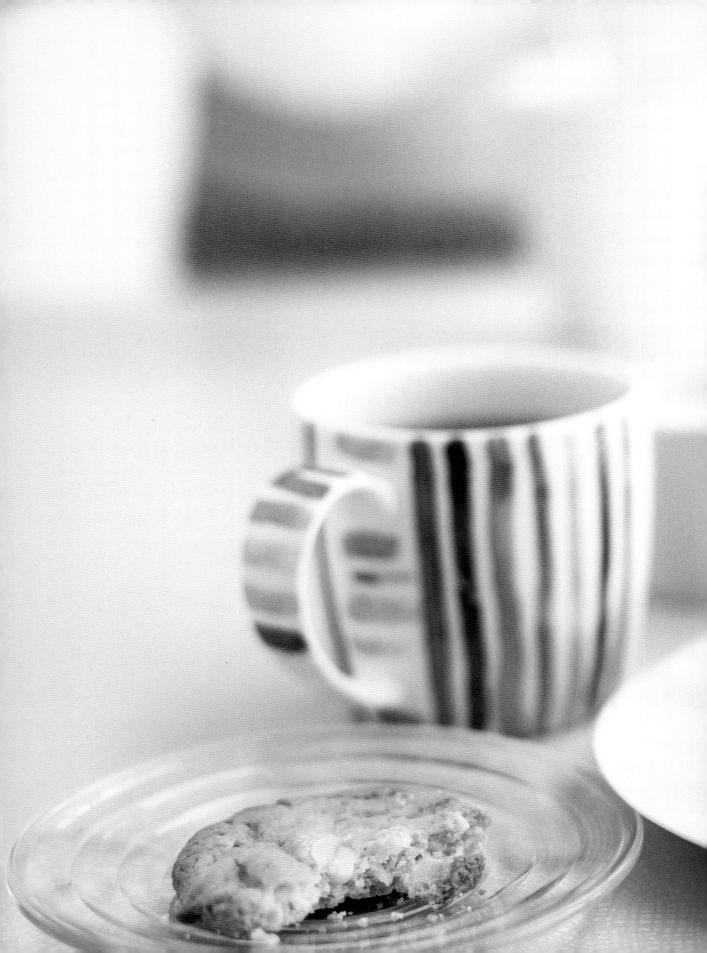

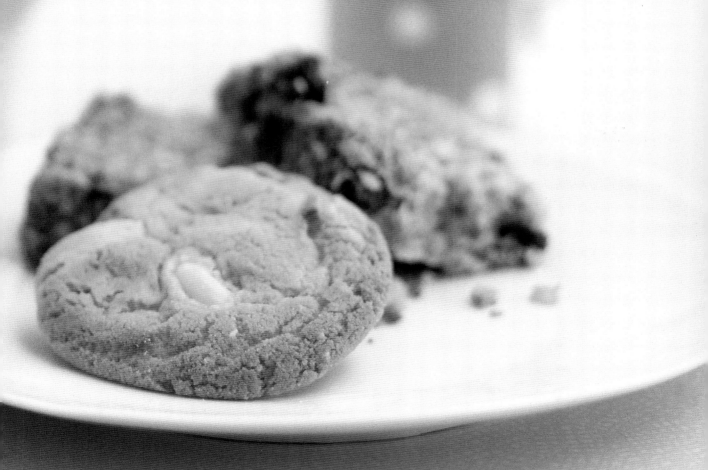

baking

preparation time
15 minutes

cooking time
15–20 minutes

makes 6 muffins

nutritional values per muffin
- 210 kcals
- 6 g fat
- 1 g saturated fat
- 1 g fiber
- Source of phytoestrogens

Cook's tip
If you don't have any apricot jam, use a little warmed marmalade instead.

carrot and orange muffins

butter, for greasing (optional)
1¼ cups (150 g) self-rising flour
½ teaspoon baking powder
⅜ cup (75 g) sugar
finely grated zest and juice of 1 orange
1 cup (about 125 g) carrots, coarsely grated
½ cup (100 ml) soy milk
2 eggs, beaten
2 tablespoons sunflower oil
1 tablespoon apricot jam, warmed

1 Line 6 muffin cups with paper bake cups or grease the cups well. Sift the flour and baking powder into a bowl and add the sugar, orange zest, and grated carrot. Mix together and make a well in the center. In a separate bowl, mix the soy milk, eggs, orange juice, and oil together. Pour the liquid into the flour and stir until just blended.

2 Fill the muffin cups two-thirds full with the mixture. Place in a preheated oven at 400°F for 15–20 minutes, or until a skewer inserted into the center comes out clean. Transfer the muffins onto a wire rack to cool.

3 Brush the tops of the muffins with a little warmed apricot jam and serve immediately.

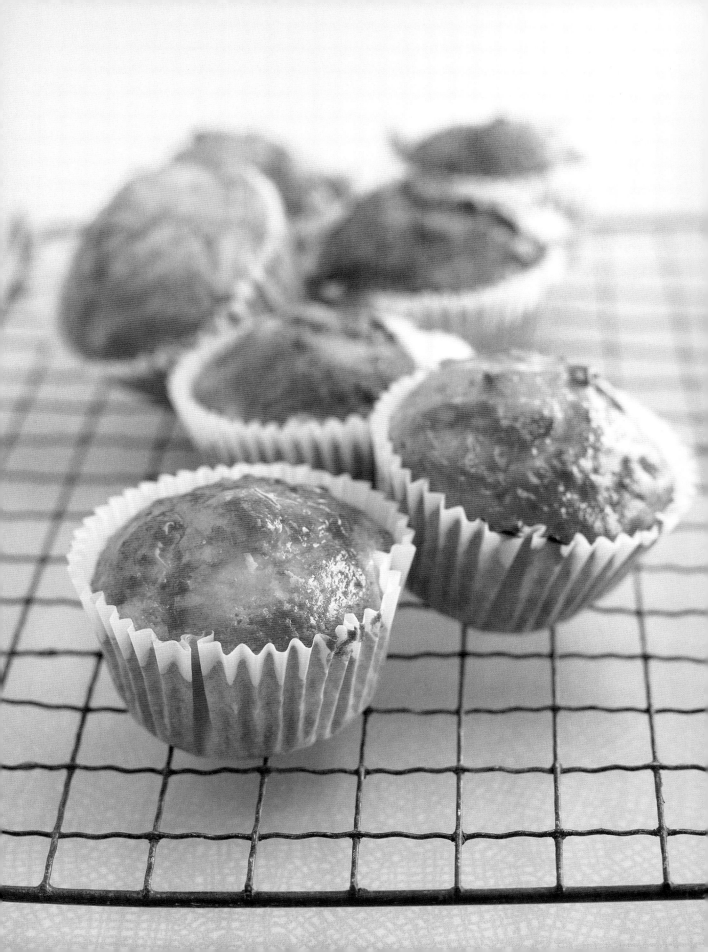

preparation time
20 minutes, plus standing

cooking time
1¼ hours

makes 2 loaves

nutritional values per slice
- 111 kcals
- 7 g fat
- 1 g saturated fat
- 2 g fiber
- Good source of phytoestrogens

fruit bread

½ cup (75 g) golden linseeds
1 cup less 2 tbsps (75 g) soy flour
1 cup (125 g) all-purpose flour
1 cup (125 g) oatmeal
⅓ cup (50 g) sunflower seeds
¼ cup (50 g) sesame seeds
½ cup (50 g) sliced almonds
1⅓ cups (200 g) golden raisins or
1½ cups (200 g) dried apricots
1 teaspoon ground cinnamon
3¼ cups (750 ml) sweetened soy milk
To decorate
1 tablespoon apricot jam, warmed
toasted sliced almonds

1 Place the linseeds in a blender or a food processor and process for 30 seconds. Alternatively, grind them in a clean coffee grinder. Place all the dry ingredients in a large bowl and mix well. Pour over the soy milk, mix again, and allow to stand for 30 minutes. If after 30 minutes the mixture seems too stiff, add a little more soy milk.

2 Line two 1-lb (500-g) loaf pans with parchment paper and spoon the mixture into the pans. Bake in a preheated oven at 375°F for about 1¼ hours, or until a skewer inserted into the center comes out clean.

3 Allow to cool in the pans for 5 minutes, then turn out onto a wire rack to cool completely. Brush with a little warmed apricot jam and decorate with toasted sliced almonds before serving.

preparation time
10 minutes, plus freezing

cooking time
15 minutes

makes about 20 crackers

nutritional values per cracker
● 80 kcals
● 5 g fat
● 2 g saturated fat
● 1 g fiber
● Source of phytoestrogens

Cook's tip
The crackers can be stored in
an airtight container for up to
1 week.

linseed crackers

3/4 cups (100 g) whole-wheat flour
3/4 cups (100 g) all-purpose flour, plus
extra for dusting
1/2 teaspoon baking powder
1/2 teaspoon baking soda
3 tablespoons golden linseeds
dash of salt
1/4 cup (50 g) butter
3 tablespoons olive oil

1 Sift the flours, baking powder, and baking soda together into a bowl, adding any bran left in the sieve. Stir in the linseeds and the salt. Cut in the butter, add the oil, and then add enough water to make a smooth dough (about 1 tablespoon should be enough).

2 Roll out the dough onto a lightly floured work surface to about 1/4 inch (5 mm) thick. Cut out rounds with a 3-in (7-cm) plain metal cookie cutter. Transfer to a lightly greased cookie sheet and bake in a preheated oven at 400°F for 15 minutes, or until golden brown. Remove from the oven. Leave to stand for 1 minute before transferring to a wire rack to cool.

preparation time
20 minutes, plus proving

cooking time
30–35 minutes

makes 2 loaves

nutritional values per slice
- 110 kcals
- 4 g fat
- 0.2 g saturated fat
- 2 g fiber
- Good source of phytoestrogens

Cook's tip
To knead the dough, stretch it away from you with the heel of your hand, then gather it up toward you. It is ready when it will stretch without breaking.

miracle bread

2^1/$_2$ cups (300 g) all-purpose flour, plus extra for dusting
3^1/$_3$ cups (350 g) whole-wheat flour
^{2}/$_3$ cup (50 g) soy flour
2 teaspoons salt
2 teaspoons fast-action dried yeast
1 teaspoon sugar
2 tablespoons sesame seeds
2 tablespoons poppyseeds
2 tablespoons golden linseeds
2 tablespoons sunflower seeds
2 tablespoons pumpkin seeds
2 cups (450 ml) warm water
1 tablespoon flaxseed oil
2 tablespoons malt extract
mixed seeds, for scattering

1 Mix the flours together in a large bowl. Stir in the remaining dry ingredients. Make a well in the center and gradually add the warm water, oil, and malt extract to form a soft dough. Turn out onto a lightly floured work surface and knead the dough for about 10 minutes, or until smooth and elastic. Return the dough to the bowl, cover with a clean, damp cloth, and leave to rise in a warm place for at least 1^1/$_2$ hours, or until doubled in size.

2 Lightly oil two 8x4x2-inch (2lb/1-kg) loaf pans. Knead the dough again, knocking out the air, then divide in half. Shape the dough into 2 loaves and press into the prepared pans. Cover loosely and allow to rise for 30 minutes, or until the dough reaches the tops of the pans.

3 Brush each loaf with a little water and scatter over a few mixed seeds. Bake in a preheated oven at 425°F for 30–35 minutes, or until risen and golden brown. Leave in the pans for 10 minutes, then transfer to a wire rack to cool.

If you prefer to make rolls, divide the mixture into 24 equal portions and place on a lightly greased cookie sheet. Bake for 15–20 minutes.

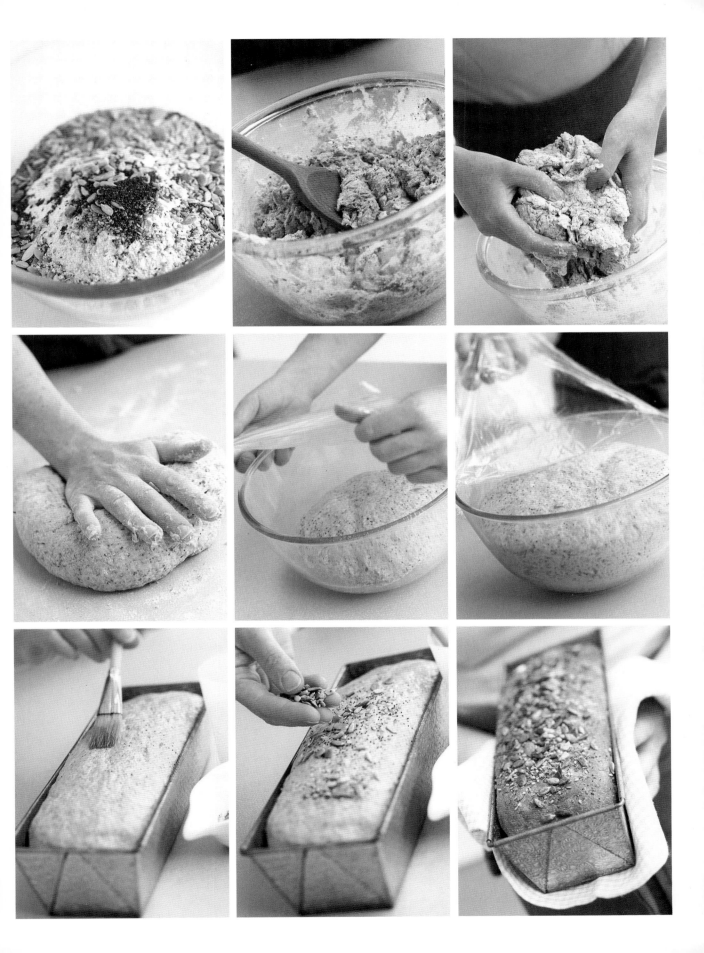

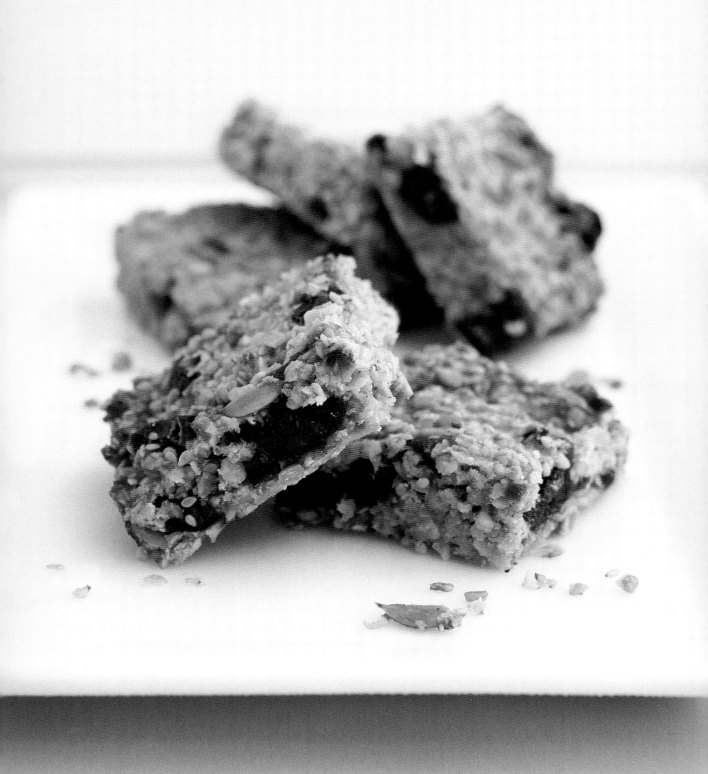

preparation time
10 minutes

cooking time
25–35 minutes

makes 9 bars

nutritional values per bar
- 250 kcals
- 15 g fat
- 7g saturated fat
- 3 g fiber
- Source of phytoestrogens

Cook's tip
Store the bars in an airtight container for up to 5 days.

banana and three-seed energy bars

½ cup (100 g) unsalted butter
3 tablespoons light corn syrup
1¼ cups (150 g) oatmeal
2 bananas, mashed (about 1 cup (250 g) in total)
½ cup (100 g) dried prunes, roughly chopped
¼ cup (25 g) pumpkin seeds
¼ cup (25 g) sunflower seeds
2 tbsp (25 g) sesame seeds

1 Lightly grease a 7-inch (18-cm) square baking pan and line the base with parchment paper. Melt the butter and syrup in a heavy saucepan until dissolved. Remove from the heat, add the remaining ingredients, and mix well.

2 Spoon the mixture into the prepared pan, level the surface, and bake in a preheated oven at 350°F for 20–30 minutes, or until golden brown. The mixture will still be very soft in the center.

3 Leave to cool in the pan for 10 minutes, then cut into 9 squares. When cold, transfer to an airtight container. Don't try to remove the bars from the pan while they are still warm because they will break.

preparation time
15 minutes

cooking time
10–15 minutes

makes about 28 cookies

nutritional values per cookie
- 122 kcals
- 7 g fat
- 3 g saturated fat
- 0.5 g fiber

peanut butter and banana cookies

1/2 cup (125 g) butter, softened
3/4 cup (150 g) sugar
1 egg, beaten
1 teaspoon baking powder
1/2 cup (125 g) crunchy peanut butter
1 1/4 cups (150 g) all-purpose flour
3 1/2 oz (100 g) dried banana chunks,
roughly chopped
28 unsalted peanuts

1 Place all the ingredients, except the banana chunks and peanuts, in a blender or food processor and process until well mixed. Stir in the banana chunks. Roll the dough into balls about the size of a walnut and place on lightly greased cookie sheets, allowing enough space for the mixture to spread as it bakes. Using the palm of your hand, flatten the balls slightly.

2 Press a whole peanut into the middle of each cookie and bake in a preheated oven at 375°F for 10–15 minutes, or until just beginning to brown around the edges.

3 Allow to cool slightly. Using a metal spatula, transfer to a wire rack to cool completely. Store in an airtight container for up to 5 days.

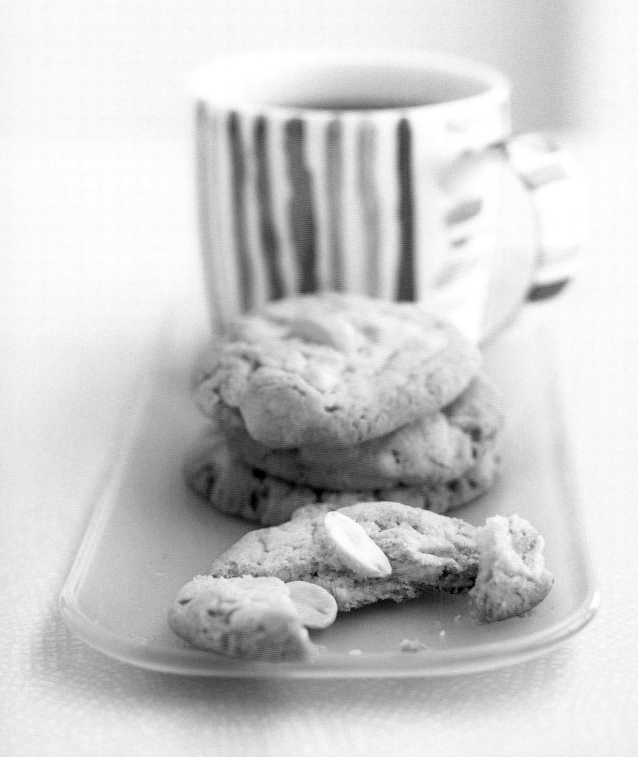

preparation time
20 minutes

cooking time
1 hour

makes 1 loaf

nutritional values per slice
- 220 kcals
- 12 g fat
- 2 g saturated fat
- 2 g fiber
- Source of phytoestrogens

banana and pumpkin bread

$^3/_4$ cup (100 g) self-rising flour
$^2/_3$ cup (75 g) whole-wheat flour
$^1/_2$ teaspoon baking soda
1 teaspoon ground cinnamon
$^1/_2$ cup (100 g) soft brown sugar
$^1/_2$ cup (100 ml) sunflower oil
4 tablespoons plain soy yogurt
2 eggs, beaten
2 cups (250 g) peeled pumpkin flesh, coarsely grated
1 banana, mashed
$^1/_3$ cup (50 g) golden raisins
$^1/_2$ cup (50 g) pecans
2 tablespoons linseeds

1 Lightly grease and line the base of an 8x4x2-inch (1-kg) loaf pan with parchment paper.

2 Sift the flours, baking soda, and cinnamon into a large bowl. Stir in the sugar. Place the oil, soy yogurt, and eggs in a separate bowl and whisk to combine. Pour the liquid into the flour and beat with an electric beater for 1 minute.

3 Stir in the pumpkin, banana, golden raisins, pecans, and linseeds and transfer the mixture to the prepared pan.

4 Bake in a preheated oven at 350°F for 1 hour, or until a skewer inserted into the center comes out clean. Allow to cool in the pan for 5–10 minutes, then carefully transfer to a wire rack to cool completely.

preparation time
20 minutes

cooking time
30–40 minutes

makes 10 slices

nutritional values per slice
- 180 kcals
- 6g fat
- 3g saturated fat
- 1g fiber
- Source of phytoestrogens

Cook's tip
The gingerbread is best left to mature for 1–2 days before eating.

gingerbread

1 cup (125 g) all-purpose flour
2/3 cup (50 g) soy flour
2 teaspoons dried ground ginger
1/2 teaspoon baking soda
1/3 cup (50 g) golden raisins
1 tablespoon preserved ginger in syrup, finely chopped
1 tablespoon linseeds
1/4 cup (50 g) butter
1/3 cup (50 g) brown sugar
1/4 cup (2 oz) light corn syrup
1/4 cup (2 oz) molasses
3 tablespoons soy milk
1 egg

1 Grease and line a 6x9-inch (15x23-cm) shallow baking pan with parchment paper. Sift the flours, dried ground ginger, and baking soda together into a bowl. Add the golden raisins, preserved ginger, and linseeds.

2 Place the butter, sugar, syrup, and molasses in a small saucepan and heat gently until melted. Add to the flour mixture together with the soy milk and the egg. Mix lightly.

3 Pour the mixture into the prepared pan. Bake in a preheated oven at 350°F for 30–40 minutes, or until a skewer inserted into the center comes out clean. Allow to cool in the pan for 5 minutes, then turn out onto a wire rack to cool completely. Store in an airtight container for up to 1 week.

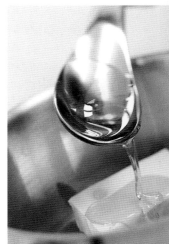

preparation time
15 minutes

cooking time
35–40 minutes

makes 10 slices

nutritional values per slice
- 136 kcals
- 2 g fat
- 2.5 g saturated fat
- 0.5 g fiber
- Source of phytoestrogens

cornbread

1 large egg
1 cup (200 ml) plain soy yogurt
2 tbsp (25 g) butter, melted
1 cup (125 g) fine cornmeal
1/2 cup (50 g) all-purpose flour
1 tablespoon baking powder
1 teaspoon salt
dash of cayenne pepper
1 large red chili, seeded and finely chopped
4 green onions, finely sliced
2/3 cup (125 g) fresh or canned sweetcorn kernels
1/2 cup (50 g) freshly grated Parmesan

1 Lightly grease and line the base of a 7-in (18-cm) square cake pan with parchment paper. Whisk the egg in a bowl until frothy, then stir in the soy yogurt and melted butter.

2 Stir in the cornmeal, flour, baking powder, salt, and cayenne pepper. Add the remaining ingredients and mix thoroughly.

3 Turn the mixture into the prepared pan and bake in a preheated oven at 350°F for 35–40 minutes, or until a skewer inserted into the center comes out clean.

4 Allow to cool in the pan for 10 minutes, then turn out onto a wire rack. When completely cold, cut into squares..

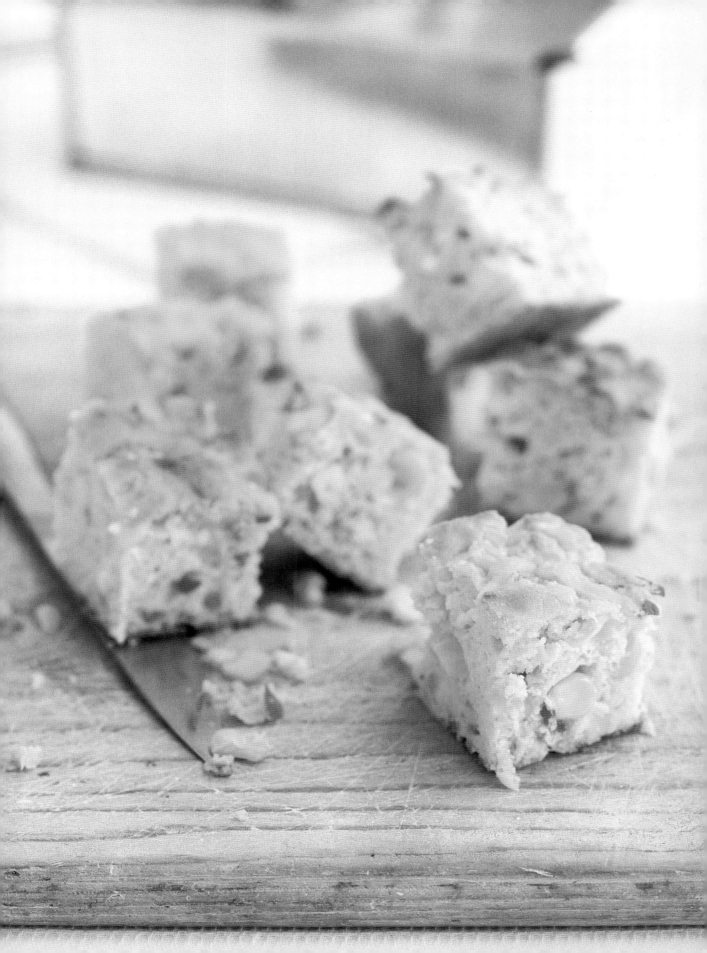

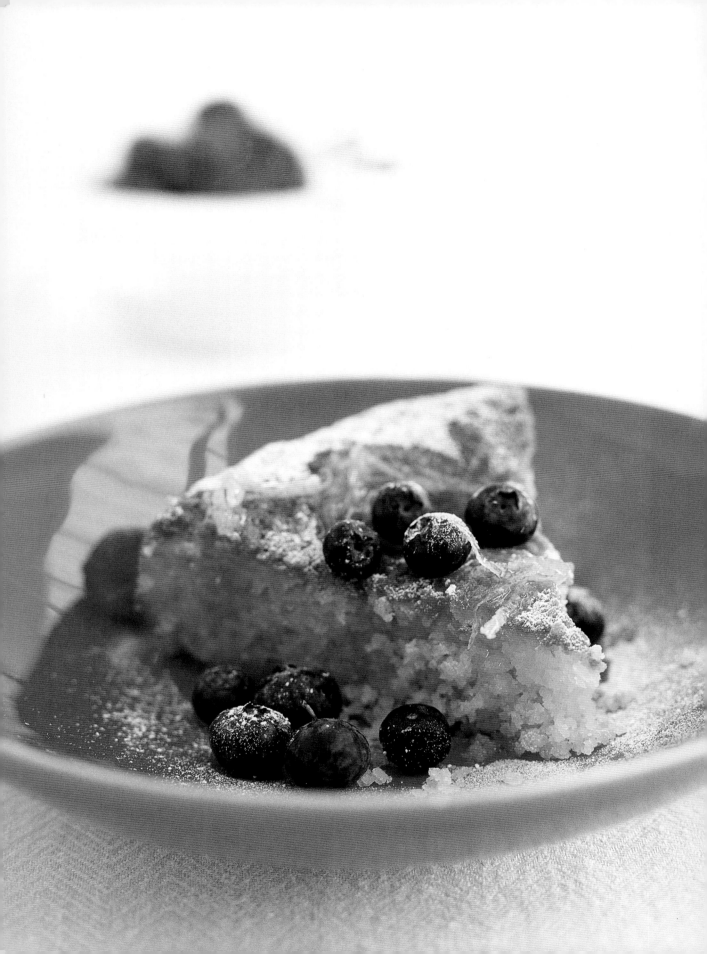

preparation time
15 minutes

cooking time
35–40 minutes

serves 8

nutritional values per serving
- 400 kcals
- 32 g fat
- 13 g saturated fat
- 2 g fiber
- Source of phytoestrogens

lemon and seed cake

¾ cup (175 g) butter
¾ cup (175 g) sugar
2 large eggs, beaten
1⅔ cups (150 g) ground almonds
½ cup (75 g) polenta or fine cornmeal
½ teaspoon baking powder
2 tablespoons linseeds
finely grated zest of 2 large lemons
2 tablespoons lemon juice
powdered sugar, to dust
raspberries or blueberries, to serve

Lemon syrup
½ cup (75 g) sugar
finely grated zest and juice of 1 large lemon
2 tablespoons water

1 Line the base of an 7-inch (18-cm) springform pan with parchment paper and lightly grease the sides. Cream the butter and sugar together in a large bowl until light and fluffy, then gradually beat in the eggs. Add the ground almonds, polenta or cornmeal, baking powder, linseeds, lemon zest, and juice and mix well.

2 Spoon the mixture into the prepared pan and bake in a preheated oven at 350°F for 35–40 minutes, or until a skewer inserted into the center comes out clean. Leave to cool in the pan.

3 To make the syrup, place all the ingredients in a small saucepan and heat until the sugar dissolves. Boil for 1 minute, then remove from the heat.

4 Remove the cake from the pan and transfer to a serving plate. Using a toothpick, prick the cake in several places. Drizzle the syrup over the cake. Dust the cake with powdered sugar and serve with fresh raspberries or blueberries.

index

a activity 22–3, 25
alcoholic drinks 13, 20, 22
antioxidants 23

b bananas 31, 33, 43, 115, 135–8
beans 13, 16, 49, 55
beans, cannellini 70, 86
beans, fava 58, 85, 89, 106
beans, mixed 61, 64, 103
beer 13
bread 19, 38, 125, 130, 132–3, 139–40
breast cancer 16
burgers 69, 103

c cakes 143
cereals 13, 16, 19, 23, 32–4
cereals, see also bread
chicken 50, 78–9
chickpeas 13, 16, 52–3, 60
cholesterol 14–15, 22–3

d dips 56–7
drinks 13, 20, 22, 40–3

e estrogen 9, 10

f fats 23
fibre 23
fish 22, 23, 49, 86–93
flax see linseeds
fruit, phytoestrogens 13, 16, 20, 23
fruit, recipes 33–7, 115–23, 130

h heart disease 10, 14–15, 22–3
Hormone Replacement Therapy (HRT) 11
hormones 9, 11
hot flashes 14, 21

HRT see Hormone Replacement Therapy
i ipriflavone 16
isoflavones 13

k kebabs 71, 98

l lentils 13, 16, 20, 65, 72, 88
lifestyle 21, 25–7
linseeds 12, 13, 16, 18, 131, 143
linseeds, see also seeds

m meat 76–85
muffins 31, 128

o osteoporosis 10, 15

p pasta 105–9
pâté 55
peas 13, 20, 66, 90
phytoestrogens 12–20
pulses see beans; chickpeas; lentils; peas

r rice 20, 79, 85, 123
rye 13, 16

s salads 47–53, 98
sauces 71, 90, 98
seeds, linseeds 12, 13, 16, 18, 131, 143
seeds, mixed 32, 48, 135
seeds, sesame 66, 78
servings 18–20
shellfish 47, 58
smoking 22
soups 63–6
soy, see also tofu
soy, benefits 14–15
soy, milk 40–3
soy, phytoestrogens 12–13, 16, 18–19, 23
soy, textured vegetable protein 18, 105

soy, yogurt 36, 115–17
supplements 16, 17, 21
symptoms 10–11, 21

t tea 20
textured vegetable protein (TVP) 18, 105
therapies 21
thyroxine 16
tofu 18, 56, 63, 69, 71, 98–102
TVP see textured vegetable protein

v vegetables 13, 16, 23
weight 23, 24–5

w wine 20

y yogurt 36, 115–17

Acknowledgments

Executive Editor Nicola Hill
Executive Art Editor Rozelle Bentheim
Editor Katy Denny
Designer Miranda Harvey
Picture Librarian Jennifer Veall
Assistant Production Controller Aileen O'Reilly
Photographer William Lingwood
Food Stylist Lucy McKelvie

Additional Photography:
Corbis UK Ltd/Rick Gomez 25 **Getty Images**/Frederic Lucano 21/Julie Toy 9 **Octopus Publishing Group Limited**/Frank Adam 12, 14 top, 18 detail 3/Colin Bowling; Organon Laboratories Ltd 11 top right; Schering Health Care Ltd 11 bottom left/Sandra Lane 17/Gary Latham 24/Peter Pugh-Cook 19 detail 1/William Reavell 14 bottom, 18 detail 2, 18 detail 5, 18 detail 6, 19 detail 5, 20 detail 4, 20 detail 5, 20 detail 6, 20 detail 7, 22/**Science Photo Library**/Sheila Terry 11 bottom right